Should Health Screening Be Private?

The IEA Health and Welfare Unit

Choice in Welfare No. 48

Should Health Screening Be Private?

Jim Thornton

IEA Health and Welfare Unit
London

First published January 1999

The IEA Health and Welfare Unit
2 Lord North St
London SW1P 3LB

ISBN 0-255 36451-2
ISSN 1362-9565

Typeset by the IEA Health and Welfare Unit

Printed in Great Britain by
St Edmundsbury Press
Bury St Edmunds, Suffolk

Contents

The Author

Jim Thornton is Reader in Obstetrics and Gynaecology at Leeds University. He qualified in medicine in Leeds in 1977 and worked for four years in Africa before training as a specialist. He has published papers on the ethics of abortion and on the problems parents face in deciding whether to undergo prenatal diagnosis. His main research consists in organising randomised controlled trials to evaluate unproven pregnancy interventions. He is also a NHS consultant at Leeds General Infirmary, involved day to day in prenatal and cervical cancer screening, and in abortion for congenital abnormality.

Foreword

Should health screening be free, or should we pay for it? Dr Jim Thornton advances a strong and scholarly argument in favour of private screening. He shows how many adult screening programmes are of questionable benefit and, in some cases, potentially harmful. The uncertainties are such that, whether a particular individual should take part in a specific screening programme, is largely a matter of personal preference. There are often no objective or scientific criteria that can be applied by doctors, and in these circumstances—though with important exceptions—the author argues that decisions should be made by patients in the light of the cost and their own values.

The author is Reader in Obstetrics and Gynaecology at Leeds University and an NHS consultant at Leeds General Infirmary, where he is involved day-to-day in prenatal and cervical cancer screening.

Few issues are more controversial, but the author's measured approach will advance understanding of the difficult choices which must be made. The IEA never expresses a corporate view in its publications but this essay by a distinguished medical practitioner can be highly recommended.

David G. Green

Acknowledgements

These ideas were first encouraged by an invitation from Lieve Christensen and her colleagues at the de Snoo van Hoogerhuis Foundation in Utrecht. Although the resulting pamphlet was too controversial for the main medical journals, David Green encouraged me to expand it into the present book. I am grateful to Mary Anderson, Kees de Boer, Lieve Christensen, David Evans, John Grant, Steve Harrison, Walter Holland, Jennifer Jackson, Nick Johnson, Terence Kealey, Maurice King, Richard Lilford, Hugh McLachlan, Mark Sculpher, Nigel Simpson, Hamish Taylor, and two anonymous referees for many helpful comments, despite some of them being out of sympathy with the ideas. Of course responsibility for the final result is mine. Finally, I thank my family for their patience during the painful process of writing this my first book.

Introduction

MOST people support health screening, because 'prevention is better than cure'. Since it works best when everyone joins in, and a free, universal, state-run scheme will usually reach more people than schemes which are private, selective or on-request, few object when the government pays. Screening tests cost a few pounds and prevent dreaded problems like cancer or brain damage. Some programmes, such as those for preventing rhesus disease, are among the most dramatic success stories of modern medicine. It is not surprising that, like motherhood and apple pie, no one is against screening.

Nevertheless, defenders of liberty should be on their guard. Funding screening through taxation is coercive. Like other forms of state coercion, it may be justified, but only for good reasons. It is wrong to argue that, since much health care is provided by the state, all of it should be. There are many reasons for state provision of health care, but they justify only a few screening programmes.

Government screening is unavoidably collectivist and the benefit and harm have to be weighed for the whole population. It is difficult to balance the disease prevented for a few against the side-effects of screening, albeit usually small, which affect many. A community cost/benefit calculation requires that the values of different people be compared. This is impossible for controversial programmes. We can never balance the value one 'pro-choice' person attaches to preventing the birth of a handicapped child against the value a 'pro-life' person attaches to preventing an abortion. For less controversial programmes interpersonal utility comparisons are possible using such techniques as the Quality Adjusted Life Year (QALY), but the methodology is not robust, and the results imprecise. No health planner can do the calculation so accurately that it can be used to override the implicit cost/benefit calculation revealed by the operation of the market.

It is also wrong to assume that health screening is so effective that people declining it must be disadvantaging themselves. All programmes have some side-effects, many are less effective than lay people often assume, and patients don't know when they take the test whether they will benefit or be harmed. Screening is a lottery. People pay a small price, if only in inconvenience and anxiety, in the hope of winning the prize of preventing serious disease. It is rational for some people to decline the lottery. Even those who recognise that there is a net benefit from screening might, if given the option, choose to spend their money on something else. Since screening uptake rates are often low among the poor, enthusiasts often characterise such people as ignorant or feckless, and take steps to coerce them to participate, such as testing when they attend for another reason. Such paternalism cannot be justified.

We should not assume that if the state did not provide it, screening would not occur. There is no reason why it should not thrive in the free market, and indeed, in places where the state refrains from getting involved, private health screening is widespread. For programmes of disputed cost/benefit, private screening would be more innovative, efficient, and responsive to individual preferences than the state. For programmes of universally agreed worth, the ability of the private sector to achieve high coverage has never been tested. However, it could respond in innovative ways, perhaps by offering cheap deals to the poor, and charities would probably fund such programmes for those who could not afford even the cheap deals. Given private sector efficiencies, coverage might even be higher than state provision. Two limited roles would remain for government. Firstly, to fill any gaps in programmes of undisputed cost/benefit for people who cannot afford them, and in particular to ensure that fetuses, children and the mentally impaired do not miss out if their parents or carers fail to arrange private testing for them. Secondly, to provide or subsidise those programmes, mainly those testing for infectious disease, which either provide a public good or have significant beneficial externalities. With these exceptions, the NHS should not screen healthy adults.

Prenatal screening where the treatment option is abortion poses special problems. Its overall worth is disputed. Decisions to fund state programmes must be based on an estimate that the lives of some people with handicap are worth less than the lives of others in full health. This is a reasonable judgement for individuals (e.g. parents) to make, but, when made by the state, it discriminates against the living handicapped. There is also a risk that state prenatal screening might one day extend to programmes to detect minor diseases, or even genes for supposed antisocial or disapproved behaviour such as homosexuality. Since prenatal screening is not a public good, and has no beneficial externalities and has these two harmful externalities (discrimination against the living handicapped, and risk of extension into eugenic programmes) it should stop. Private prenatal testing will also sometimes result in parents choosing to abort their pregnancies for reasons of which other people disapprove. Nevertheless it should be permitted, if abortion in general is permitted.

In chapter one I briefly describe the principles and scope of health screening. In chapter two I describe the major justifications which have been advanced for state intervention in health care, the harm of government health intervention, and draw attention to the special harm from government prenatal screening involving abortion. In chapter three I examine how these arguments apply to specific screening programmes. In chapter four I describe some real examples of private screening initiatives, and in chapter five I look at the political implications, and make recommendations for action.

This book might be perceived to be an attack on screening. It is not. It is a criticism of government screening. I am an enthusiast for screening and professionally engaged in supplying it. I believe there is scope for more screening, but only if it is efficient and sensitive to consumer demand. This can usually best be achieved privately. Similarly the discussion of prenatal screening might be construed as anti-abortion. Nothing could be further from the truth. I am 'pro-choice', involved daily in prenatal diagnosis, and as a gynaecologist perform abortions. However, some people of goodwill regard abortion as morally equivalent to murder and object to paying, via their taxes, for screening programmes that encourage it. This is different from objecting to taxation to fund the army or the police. It is reasonable to force people to contribute to those goods which otherwise would not exist, and from which everyone benefits. No such reasons justify most government screening.

1

Introduction to Health Screening

SCREENING is the testing of apparently healthy individuals for disease or its precursors, so that early and more effective treatment may be given. In recent years it has grown into a major part of the health care enterprise, which in most countries is paid for by the state. In the UK, general practitioners are each paid about £2,000 per annum to encourage them to screen their patients, participation in some programmes is now a contractual obligation, and there is both lay and professional encouragement to increase NHS screening activity.

Screening differs from traditional medicine in that it does not arise from a patient's request for advice for a specific complaint. This means that people offering it should be particularly careful to ensure that they have good evidence that, taking everything into account, the programme is worthwhile. This is surprisingly difficult to demonstrate, as is evidenced by the repeated efforts of experts to draw up lists of the conditions necessary for a successful programme (Wilson and Jungner 1968, Cuckle and Wald 1984, Holland and Stewart 1990). The disease must be an important health problem, doctors must have a reasonable understanding of the biology, there must be a recognisable early stage to the disease, and treatment at this early stage must be of more benefit than treatment started later. Both the tests and the treatment must be acceptable to people. Finally the gain should outweigh the harm by a sufficient margin to make the screening more worthwhile than alternative uses to which the money might have been put. Usually, only the individual involved can decide whether the tests are acceptable, and whether the gain outweighs the harm, since only they know their personal preferences and values. However, if the state is to provide a programme, it must somehow calculate that the screening is worthwhile to society as a whole.

This is sometimes possible for programmes with clear-cut benefit and trivial harm. For programmes with disputed benefit or significant harm it would mean overriding the values of some people. It is also noteworthy that none of these descriptions of the criteria required for a successful programme include any reasons why the screening should be provided by the state, as opposed to privately.

Types of Screening

There are two ways to organise screening: centrally planned or consumer-led. Most public health specialists argue that centrally planned programmes are preferable, because they can be limited to those that experts think are worthwhile, they may achieve higher uptake, and they can be focused on the groups at highest risk. It is argued that consumer-led programmes are inferior, because they include screening tests of unproven effectiveness and those of which experts disapprove. Consumer-led programmes may start before facilities for diagnosis and treatment are fully established, and typically people attending such programmes tend to be healthier, and supposedly in less need of screening, than those who do not (Hart 1971). However, consumer-led screening has the advantage that, in general, it only includes programmes that the people who undergo it think are worthwhile, and people who do not want to be screened do not feel pressurised to accept. If privately run, such programmes typically include a battery of screening tests at a single visit, which increases efficiency.

In a classical screening programme, whether public or private, the provider waylays healthy people outside the health care arena, either by advertising or by written invitations. This is intrusive, particularly if the invitation alerts people to a risk of disease of which they were unaware. An alternative is case-finding, or opportunistic screening. Here patients who consult a doctor for another reason are offered a screening test at the same time. Much of prenatal screening is like this. Other examples include offering cervical smears to women asking for contraceptive advice, or testing for cystic fibrosis carrier status, or measuring blood pressure, when people attend for an unrelated problem. Case-finding is attractive to screeners since it is cheap to organise and often achieves high uptake, especially among the poor and deprived, who typically have low attendance rates for conventional screening. The disadvantages are that the ease of introducing case-finding means that it may displace other worthwhile activity, and facilities for quality control, and for diagnosis and treatment of identified abnormalities, may not be in place. More importantly, patients may permit themselves to be tested without really wanting it. They may want to please the doctor, be too ill to resist, or mistakenly think that the test is to sort out the problem they came with, rather than to look for an unrelated one. Of course private screening programmes also persuade people by advertising but this is usually much easier to resist than a doctor's apparently impartial advice. In the long run, programmes that depend on heavy advertising will be relatively unprofitable and providers will direct their energies elsewhere.

The Benefit and Harm of Screening

The benefit of screening can be considerable. It mainly accrues to those people who were destined to develop a serious disease, but who were detected by the screening programme early enough for successful prevention or cure. In addition, those who would have been cured anyway when the disease presented naturally might benefit from less radical treatment, and people with negative results might benefit from the reassurance.

Nevertheless, the harm is easily underestimated. It is obvious that those who have a false positive screening test, and undergo unnecessary further testing or treatment, are harmed. They will be made anxious (Cuckburn *et al* 1994), and may also be physically harmed. Even people with a true positive result may be harmed if they were not ultimately destined to develop the disease; not all people carrying an abnormal gene go on to have affected children. People with a disease will have a longer period of morbidity the earlier it is diagnosed. Although this may be outweighed by the benefit of early diagnosis if treatment is effective, it is still a harm. There are also direct hazards from the screening test itself. Even a blood test is painful and causes bruising, and all women find cervical smears at least mildly unpleasant. Mammography involves a small dose of radiation and many patients find the manipulation painful and distressing. People with a false negative result will be falsely reassured, and even those with a true negative result might engage in less healthy behaviour as a result (Tymstra and Bielman 1987, Stewart-Brown and Farmer 1997). It has even been claimed that screening programmes cause people to have a reduced sense of personal control over health, poorer self-rated health, more episodes of illness and less self-initiated preventive care (Seeman and Seeman 1983, Stewart-Brown and Farmer 1997). Finally, there are resource costs. People take time off work to be screened and time spent screening by medical staff is time not spent dealing with clinical problems.

Personal Values and Screening

The decision to undergo a screening test is no different from any other decision in medicine. It has to be made under conditions of uncertainty because we cannot know the future. It is a lottery ticket that costs a small amount of anxiety and inconvenience, and most people win nothing. A few people win a lot if they have their cancer, stroke or handicapped child's birth prevented. Nevertheless, there are still good and bad decisions. Good decisions take account of both the chances of each outcome, and of the values (utility) the decision-maker attaches to them. Generally a good decision maximises the product of these, expected utility. If everyone agrees on the values to be used, the decision may appear to be unaffected by personal values, but this is an illusion. Consider the decision to undergo surgery for appendicitis. Surgeons do not usually discuss whether patients wish to take a risk of dying to avoid an abdominal scar. They simply tell patients whether, in their judgement, surgery or observation is the safest option, and proceed accordingly. People value avoiding a scar on their abdomen as trivial compared with dying, and since not operating on appendicitis has significant mortality, the decision is easy. Nevertheless a value judgement has been made in that case. Even an abdominal scar is a measurable harm. If a million people had to undergo one, to save one life, we might decide to avoid surgery. Some people might value an abdominal scar differently to others. Glamour models are presumably keen to avoid them.

Sometimes people's differing values make a crucial difference to the right decision. Prenatal diagnosis is a good example. Sometimes parents learn that there is a risk that their unborn baby has an abnormality, say spina bifida, which is associated with severe handicap, in this case problems with walking and bladder control. If it could be diagnosed, the parents might wish to abort the pregnancy. However, the diagnosis is not certain and a further test, amniocentesis, is required. This involves passing a needle into the womb. It will give a clear result, but carries a risk of causing miscarriage. Let us assume that the risk of spina bifida is one in 200 (0.5 per cent) and that the risk of the needle causing miscarriage is one in 100 (one per cent). The correct course of action is not obvious. It depends on how the parents feel about having a handicapped child and about abortion. Some parents feel that having a handicapped child would be terrible, but would not be devastated by abortion. Perhaps they have plenty of children already, or the pregnancy was an accident. They would probably choose to undergo the test, and might even undergo it at much lower risks of handicap. Other parents might feel that handicap, while unfortunate, was not the worst that could happen, that such children often led very worthwhile lives, and that overcoming handicap can be quite life-enhancing. For yet a third group of parents the pregnancy might be very precious, especially if they had suffered prolonged infertility. Both these latter groups of parents might well decline amniocentesis unless the risk of spina bifida was much higher. Parents who were opposed to abortion for religious reasons would probably never choose amniocentesis at all. All the parents, making different decisions given the same probabilities, would be making correct decisions. The reason is that their values differ.

Personal values affect screening decisions in similar ways. Often screening has a relatively trivial harm, but many people undergo it, and value it differently. For example, some might reckon that it is worth a hundred mammograms to save one life, others might reckon it is worth a thousand. At other times only a few may suffer a substantial harm, but again may value it differently. For example, some might reckon that it is worth making five middle-aged men impotent to save one life, and others that it is worth 50.

Measuring the Cost/Benefit Ratio of Screening

This is always difficult, even for individuals; for populations it is often impossible (Drummond *et al* 1987). The costs are difficult to calculate because they not only include both the direct costs of the programme and the indirect costs such as those to the patient in time off work etc., but also need to take account of the timing of costs and benefits. Most costs from a screening programme occur now, while the benefits are delayed and should be discounted. Measuring the net benefit of a screening programme is even more difficult than measuring the costs. Even if we know the effectiveness of a programme in, say, reducing mortality, we need to measure the harms on the same scale, to calculate overall utility. This involves measuring the value of life or health of different individuals. Normally this cannot be done. I cannot say whether my life is worth more or less to me than your life is worth to you. We can only compare different people's values if everyone agrees on the scale to use. Sometimes they do. People will often accept that a year of life is of equal worth to everyone. We can then say for example that kidney transplants cost £17,000 per life-year gained, cervical cancer screening £9,000 and breast cancer screening £8,000 (Working Group on Acute Purchasing 1996). If we accept such calculations, it is better to spend available resources on breast cancer screening than kidney transplants, assuming we cannot afford both. If different interventions improve quality of life as well, things get more complicated, but so long as everyone agrees that one year of life for one individual counts one, and death always counts zero, we can place intermediate health states on this scale, and sum utility for different individuals. The quality adjusted life-year (QALY) is a popular way of putting different health states on the same scale (Rosser *et al* 1982, Sackett and Torrance 1978, Maynard 1991) although the practical difficulties are considerable (Mason *et al* 1993). This is called a cost/utility analysis.

However, for controversial programmes such as those involving abortion, agreement even on the scale to use is impossible. It is not only difficult to weigh up the harm that accrues to one individual against the benefit that accrues to another, but logically impossible (Arrow 1963a). No amount of careful calculation will ever enable us to measure the overall utility of a programme involving abortion. Imagine if one person claimed that abortion for her was a thousand times worse than birth of a handicapped child, and a hundred other people said that for them the birth of a handicapped child was twice as bad as abortion. In economic jargon there is no population-utility function.

Even for less controversial programmes, a cost/utility analysis that weighs the medical benefits and harms precisely is inadequate for deciding whether the programme should take place at all. That requires that the net benefit of the programme be weighed against the net benefits of the other uses to which the money could be put, including non-health care uses. People may agree that a screening programme produces more utility per pound than other health interventions, but still feel that they would get more benefit from spending the money on education, law and order, or a holiday. To decide whether to spend money on a screening programme at all, we need to measure its benefit on a universal scale, against which other activities can also be measured. The only realistic scale is money itself.

There are two ways to use money to perform a cost/benefit analysis. The ideal is to observe people's spending decisions. People take account of all their other priorities when they spend their own money, and providers respond to the demand resulting from their decisions by diverting resources appropriately. This makes the market price for a good a finely calibrated and flexible method for indicating preferences across a wide range of choices. Unfortunately, since the state already provides most health care in this country, the market is distorted, and opportunities for observing people's health care purchasing are limited. Nevertheless, the fact that some people pay for, say, hip replacement, and that most private insurance packages cover this operation, confirms that hip replacement is cost/beneficial, at least to those individuals who take out insurance. The opposite observation, failure of people to buy or take out insurance to cover a service already provided by the state, does not necessarily indicate that the service is not cost/beneficial. We can say only that state provision is adequate, but not whether it is optimal or excessive. However, if a health intervention is not provided by the state and no one buys it, e.g. screening for toxoplasmosis infection in pregnancy, we can be confident that it is not cost/beneficial (Thornton 1994).

In the absence of a health care market, an inferior alternative is to measure people's hypothetical 'willingness to pay'. This involves asking people how much they would be willing to pay for a service if they became ill, or more realistically how much they would pay as an insurance premium, so that it was available when needed. Published experience with this kind of exercise is limited (Berwick and Weinstein 1985, Donaldson 1990) and people may overstate their real willingness to pay. Nevertheless, if an intervention costs more than a person's stated willingness to pay it cannot be cost/beneficial for that individual. If it costs more than even wealthy people's stated willingness to pay it cannot be cost/beneficial for less wealthy people.

To summarise, it is impossible to measure the cost/benefit ratio of any screening programme, unless people agree on their aims and priorities. This means that health planners cannot objectively measure the cost/benefit of any disputed screening programme without overriding the values of some individuals. The best they can do is observe free agents buying screening, or taking out insurance to cover it, in a free market.

The Scope of Screening

The UK National Health Service (NHS)

The NHS runs three systematic national programmes in which healthy adults are invited for screening, namely hypertension, cervical cytology and mammography. Parents are also offered a new-born screen for their children, which as a minimum includes a physical examination, a test for congenital dislocation of the hip, and a blood test for phenylketonuria and hypothyroidism. Older children are screened for dental disease, incomplete immunisation status, impaired vision and hearing, and for delayed development, on a number of occasions in childhood and adolescence. All pregnant women are offered some form of prenatal care. This always includes screening for anaemia, diabetes, syphilis, rhesus disease, and hypertension, and the offer of an ultrasound examination of the fetus to test for a range of structural abnormalities, including spina bifida. Screening for Down's syndrome is usually offered to older women, although the age cut-off varies. A lot of other NHS screening goes on. This is mainly opportunistic screening of high risk groups, or general screening to limited populations because of local initiatives, pilot studies or research. All the above NHS screening is free.

Private

The screening offered in the private health care system varies between companies, but the British United Provident Association (BUPA) offers hypertension, cholesterol, thyroid, electrocardiogram, lung function, faecal occult blood, urine analysis, mammography, cervical cytology, and prostate specific antigen testing. In contrast to NHS screening, these are generally offered as part of a package. The full BUPA health screening package for adults, consisting of all these tests as appropriate, costs £340 for men and £360 for women. A limited heart screen package of blood pressure, height, weight, urine, electrocardiogram, and cholesterol costs £160, a limited well woman package of cervical smear, pelvic exam, breast self exam, blood pressure, cholesterol and rubella costs £165, or £125 without mammography, while a mammogram alone costs £85. Other private companies have similar charges to BUPA, but some independent charities subsidise their screening work and charge significantly less. The Marie Stopes clinics for example charge £55 for a well woman examination excluding mammography, and £55 for a well man examination excluding prostate specific antigen testing. BUPA does not offer pregnancy screening for congenital abnormality where the main treatment option is likely to be abortion, such as Down's syndrome and spina bifida. However, at least two other companies offer this service privately in the UK, at a cost for Down's screening of between £50 and £100 per test.

2

Why Should the State Fund Health Care in General?

Introduction

THE United Kingdom National Health Service provides medical care to all, regardless of the ability to pay, funded from general taxation, and mainly free at the point of delivery. It is so much part of the fabric of life in the UK, that it is easy to forget that there is no automatic reason to provide health care in this way. If the NHS had never existed, health care would still be provided privately and by charities, albeit in a different way or to a different extent. There may be advantages to paying for some health care from taxation, but there are also reasons of principle and of expedience to limit it as far as possible. Taxation is coercive. Democratic governments can force people to pay for almost anything so long as a majority of voters can be induced to support it. Nevertheless, governments limit freedom as they do so, and should have good moral reasons to justify such action. The self-interest, even of the majority, is not sufficient. It is also expedient to limit government intervention as far as possible since it tends to be both less sensitive to consumer preferences and less efficient than the free market. The onus of proof should therefore be on those who argue for free state provision.

The Advantages of State Funding

Three arguments are often used to justify government provision of health care. The first has intuitive appeal, but little philosophical base, and its practical application is limited. It is the idea that health care is a special need the state should provide for everyone, rather that a want, which people should choose for themselves. Many attempts have been made to define needs but none provide a clear guide for action. The second reason given for state intervention in health care is to improve equity or justice. This is more intellectually respectable, but has limited applicability to health screening because the benefit of so much screening is disputed. If we cannot agree that something is a benefit, supplying it to poor people is a bad way to correct injustice. Finally, there are economic reasons for state intervention, namely that health care should be supplied by the state, in so far as this provides a public good, increases beneficial externalities, reduces harmful externalities, or corrects market failure.

Wants and Needs

People want many things, but that does not mean that other people should be forced to supply them. However, some wants are so important that people need them for a reasonable life. It is claimed that other people (the state) should supply such needs to those who otherwise would not be able or willing to pay for them. Unfortunately it is difficult to define a need, and economists generally do not recognise the distinction. Nevertheless, like elephants, most people recognise needs when they see them. Staple food, warm clothing and basic shelter are needs. Everybody needs them to live a fulfilled life, whatever their personal priorities for other things. Exotic food, designer clothes and large houses are wants. Some people want them, but others regard them as relatively unimportant, and it is possible to live a fulfilled life without them.

Not all health care is a need. It is clear from people's behaviour that, as far as their own health goes, it is important but not an absolute priority. If it were, no one would smoke, drink, be sexually promiscuous, climb mountains or drive their car too fast. The question is what sort of health care should be classified as a need? Most curative medicine for acute illness, such as treatment of pneumonia, the setting of broken bones, or the relief of pain, are needs. Without them people either die or cannot live a decent life. In contrast homeopathy, cosmetic surgery, psychoanalysis, and spa treatment for minor illnesses are wants. Most people prefer to spend their money on other things, and live perfectly satisfactory lives without any of them, and no one ever died from the lack of them. Unfortunately clear cut cases like these do not help us decide about disputed health interventions. For this we need a definition of need. A number have been offered.

The Social Contract

It is often claimed that needs arise out of a social contract. 'Needs' consist of those things which it 'goes without saying' we must have, and which we can legitimately expect others in the community to provide if we lack them. Clearly there will be debate about what sort of health care 'goes without saying' but we can often agree on what is excluded by this definition. If, in the absence of state provision, the average person would not take out insurance cover for a health intervention, it hardly 'goes without saying' that it is a need which the state should supply. This is Dworkin's 'prudent insurer' principle (Dworkin 1995). Since screening is generally cheap and not paid for out of insurance, the test for screening should be whether, in the absence of state provision, the average prudent person would pay for it. Those screening programmes whose benefit is disputed are clearly wants.

Clinical Need

Doctors define clinical need. This is superficially attractive because of doctors' scientific knowledge and practical, albeit second-hand, experience of illness. Unfortunately it is not helpful in disputed cases, because doctors disagree. This hardly inspires confidence, and most people are unwilling to leave such important decisions to one expert group, particularly when what they consider a need seems to vary, depending how they are paid. Relatively little of modern medicine is mandated by objective clinical justification. Most of it follows patient preferences and judgements and is more like a want (Devlin *et al* 1990).

Capacity to Benefit

Some health planners define need for an intervention as simply the capacity to benefit from it (Culyer 1998). A person may be very ill, but, if it is not possible for the intervention to help him or her, there is no need for it. This is reasonable but on its own does not move us very far forward. If we cannot provide for all needs we require some measure of capacity to benefit. There are immense practical difficulties in measuring this even for curative interventions, and scales such as the quality adjusted life-year (QALY, see p. 10) have to be invoked (Maynard 1991). For disputed interventions such as screening, where the question is not just which health intervention to choose, but whether to spend our money on health screening at all or on something else entirely, we need to measure benefit on a universal scale; either money itself or 'willingness to pay'. This leads us back to arguing that screening is not cost/ beneficial unless the prudent person would pay for it.

Needs and Ethical Imperatives

Most people feel that they cannot stand idly by when an identified person's life is in danger. If rescue requires an expensive or complicated treatment that only the state can provide, then the state must do so, without worrying about the cost. This is 'the rule of rescue' (Hadorn 1991). The ethical imperative defines the need. Although it may seem to commit us to the impossible, the rule of rescue is a good rule to live by. Individuals who follow it, and societies which inculcate it in their children, generally do better than those which do not. The father of a child dying for lack of an expensive operation is right to move heaven and earth to get treatment for her. However, it does not commit us to fund screening. By definition, screening is the identification of disease of which the sufferer is unaware. There is no identified person to rescue.

Population Need

Populations can have needs. If one group has a higher mortality than another, and the difference can be attributed to lack of a particular health intervention, we can argue that the population has a need for that intervention. If there is no attributable difference between the populations despite a difference in the availability of the health intervention, then we would label the intervention a want. Again there will be debate over what population differences are relevant, but this way of thinking indicates that ineffective health care and health care of disputed overall benefit are clearly wants. For example, an intervention would only be classified as meeting a need if the lack of it was actually causing the worse health outcomes in the deprived population. People are not deprived by the lack of a screening programme that does not actually improve health, however much they may want it.

In summary, health screening is only a want, unless the average prudent person would pay for it in a private health care system. The fact that doctors say it is a clinical need is no argument. If a screening programme could be shown to be the most cost/beneficial way to spend money, health planners would regard it as a need. Again, they could only show this if the average prudent person would pay for it. Health screening is never a need according to the 'rule of rescue'. Populations can only be said to need a health intervention if a difference in health results from lack of the intervention.

Equity

In general the poor suffer disproportionately from ill health, and in private systems receive disproportionately little health care, particularly expensive interventions. If the state gives them free health care it redresses some of the inequality. However, the state is not justified in trying to correct all inequalities. It should leave alone those that cannot be corrected, and those that result from individuals' free choice. This leads us back to whether health screening is really beneficial or not, and whether it is a want or a need. Remember that the benefits of screening are not available without the side-effects. What is available is a lottery ticket which costs money, anxiety and inconvenience, but which might result in a big win—the prevention of serious disease. If the average prudent person does not buy such a screening lottery ticket, giving more tickets to the poor will not correct the inequality. It would be better to give them the money the screening would cost. If it is only a want, such that many people would prefer a holiday or better food, differential uptake simply means the poor have other priorities. Again, it would be better to give them the money. This particularly applies to expensive screening programmes. Imagine one that cost £200 per person screened, or say £20,000 per life-year gained. Even if there were no inconveniences or side-effects, many people would choose to spend their money elsewhere. The state should let them do so.

Some readers will balk at the possibility of adult poor people getting less effective screening than the rich in private systems. Let me spell out again why this is acceptable. Screening is a want not a need. The evidence is that many rich people, who could well have afforded to, did not pay for screening programmes before the NHS started providing them, and many even now do not pay for those the NHS does not yet provide. For example, I myself, a well-off consultant, would not spend my own money on any of the currently available adult health screening programmes. If we accept that screening is a want we should not be concerned if the poor undergo less of it than the rich. To worry about them getting less screening is no more logical than worrying about them taking fewer holidays in the Bahamas, or drinking less freshly-squeezed orange juice! In fact we should be more concerned at both the latter inequities because holidaying in the Bahamas and drinking fresh orange juice are more universally agreed to be components of the good life than health screening. Since the overall worth of so much screening is disputed, the poor may even benefit by getting less.

Screening For Children

Giving people free health care, which they would not buy for themselves if they were given the money instead, is patronising unless health planners know people's priorities better than they do themselves. This is not true of the adult poor, but may apply to children and the handicapped. Normally the care of children is best left to those with the most interest in their welfare, their parents. They choose how much money to spend on their food, education, health or entertainment, and can generally be trusted to do the best for the child. The advantages are that diversity and responsibility are encouraged and parents work harder for their own children than they would for children in general. Decisions about screening should therefore be left to parents. Nevertheless, it is unfair to leave children to the mercy of lazy, feckless or ignorant parents, and the state is justified in providing at least a minimum level of health and education for such children. Similar arguments apply to other vulnerable groups such as the mentally handicapped. Government provision of effective screening for children and the handicapped may be justified when a similar programme for healthy adults would not.

Economic Reasons For State Provision

Three economic reasons are usually offered for state provision of health: the correction of market failure, the provision of public goods and the improvement of externalities (Arrow 1963b, Diamond 1992).

Market Failure

Market failure can arise in insurance-based health care. Private insurance systems have two main problems: 'adverse selection' and 'moral hazard'. Adverse selection is the process whereby sick individuals tend to buy more insurance and use it more, leading insurers to either exclude such customers or charge them more. This makes health care difficult for the sick to obtain, and the defensive efforts by insurers to identify high risk customers put up health costs without improving outcomes. Moral hazards are the processes whereby insured individuals tend to use more health care as its marginal cost to them is reduced, providers encourage unnecessary treatment if neither they nor the customer are paying, and people take less care of themselves knowing that others will pay the bills. Privately funded screening is affected by neither problem. It is so cheap that it does not need to be insurance-based, so there is little risk of adverse selection, and there is no moral hazard. Moral hazard is created by state provision. For example, a person who valued a screening test below the market rate would not buy private testing, but if it was worth anything at all to them, would accept free state testing. As someone once said: 'If it's free, I'll take two.'

Market failure will also arise in cash-based systems if individuals lack the information to make an informed choice. However, this rarely justifies free state provision. If individuals are under-informed of the benefits of a health care intervention, the market will rapidly correct this by advertising. If they are under-informed of the adverse effects so that uptake is too high, it could be argued that the state should provide the missing information, but it would make no sense for the state to provide the intervention free.

Some people may be concerned at the encouragement of ineffective screening by commercial interests, and occasionally argue for regulation or banning of such tests on the grounds that customers are unaware of their ineffectiveness. The only justification for this would be if such tests harmed third parties. The state is no more justified in restricting peoples freedom to waste their own money on screening than on any other activity which harms no one else. In practice, waste on ineffective screening tests is insignificant compared with the waste on ineffective alternative medicine or skin care.

Public Goods and Externalities

Public goods are products or services from which individuals benefit without limiting others' use of them. They are under provided in private markets because it is difficult to find anyone altruistic enough to pay for them. An example would be mosquito control programmes to prevent malaria. Externalities are spill-over benefits and harms that do not affect the individual decision-maker. An example of a beneficial externality would be the reduction in transmission of sexually transmitted disease from treatment of asymptomatic infection. Since the individual reaps little or no benefit for themselves, such treatment will be priced too high in private markets. A harmful externality would be the development of antibiotic resistance from widespread use.

The provision of public goods, the maximisation of beneficial externalities and reduction of harmful ones, justify much state health intervention, but not screening. Screening is not a public good. There are plenty of incentives for private provision. Similarly, there are rarely significant beneficial externalities. The benefit affects the individual decision-maker and is therefore weighed in the balance by that person. An exception is screening for infectious diseases. The unscreened population who avoid infection because some people have been screened and treated benefit from the screening without paying for it. With one exception, there are few harmful externalities from most screening. The exception is prenatal screening for abortion, which may cause the living handicapped to feel undervalued, or develop into a eugenic programme that is unjust to unpopular minorities. These externalities are discussed below. Preventing orphans by stopping mothers dying of cervical cancer is not an externality, because the women themselves can weigh this risk in the balance when they decide about screening.

Of course the resources used to treat screen-positive patients are externalities if the state provides them free. The general public find themselves paying for diagnostic tests and treatments because someone decided to undergo a screening test, and it could be argued that the state is therefore justified in restricting people's freedom to spend money on such tests. However, this problem affects many activities and is not generally regarded as a reason to discourage people participating in those activities. Alpine climbers take greater risks knowing that mountain rescue and orthopaedic care are free, and motorists drive faster knowing that if needed a free ambulance will arrive within minutes to take them to casualty. If the NHS treats them the same as it treats patients with a disease for which they bear no responsibility, it should also treat people the same who have increased their treatment costs by well meaning attempts to improve their health.

Summary

The economic decision maker would argue that health screening is not a public good, but the state may be justified in providing it if it has a beneficial externality which would result in private screening being overpriced. The ethical decision maker would provide effective screening on grounds of equity to children and the handicapped, but not try to correct inequity by paying for free screening for the poor, especially if there is evidence that if given the choice they would spend the money elsewhere.

The Disadvantages of State Funding

Restriction of Liberty

Unlike private concerns, which obtain their money by voluntary exchange, no one gives money to the state voluntarily. Governments obtain it by the threat of force. We call it taxation. This restricts liberty since the options of citizens to spend their money elsewhere are removed. If a health intervention is provided free, everyone is forced to pay for it. This causes resentment if the service is not universally agreed to be worthwhile. Cosmetic surgery and tattoo removal are obvious examples of treatments which are unobjectionable when provided privately, but hotly debated when funded publicly.

Loss of Market Price Signals

Governments are generally less sensitive to consumers' wishes than private concerns, being more likely to respond to political signals from the electorate and pressure groups. Compared with the information contained in free market prices, these are crude. Elections occur only every four or five years and are usually decided on the basis of a small number of 'headline' issues. The signals from pressure groups are slightly less crude, but are also often misleading, in that the well organised and vocal tend to be over represented. Of course the government responds to market signals in its everyday decisions, but, insofar as the government interferes with resource allocation, it also distorts them.

This lack of health care price signals makes it difficult for providers to allocate public health resources, and leads to insoluble debates about priorities. The professionals who conduct such debates are called health economists. They have failed to answer the most basic resource allocation questions, and cannot even tell us whether overall health funding is too high or too low. Without a real health care market they have no measure of people's real preferences, or of how much health care a free market would supply. The only reliable measures of value derive from sectors, such as the pharmaceutical industry, still in private hands, and even these have been distorted by government interference (Green *et al* 1997). The lack of market price information is particularly important in areas of disputed benefit such as screening. Attempts to work out the costs of procedures in artificial markets such as the NHS internal market have failed because of the inability to measure cross-subsidies and the absence of market discipline.

Inefficiency

Governments are generally less efficient than private providers because they lack the discipline of competition and bankruptcy, and the inefficiencies of the NHS are part of everyday experience in the UK. The long-standing 'personal view' series in the *British Medical Journal* in which patients and doctors report their experiences of illness provides many examples, including, brutal and uncaring doctors (Anonymous 1995b, and 1997), dehumanising of patients (Reynolds 1996), bureaucracy gone mad (Wenham 1996), clinical incompetence (Mansley 1996), decrepit buildings

(Britchford 1996), and general inefficiency (Jackoby and McCann 1995, Juniper 1996). Such reports ring true and are presumably only the tip of an iceberg. They would not be tolerated in the private sector. Senior staff are not immune. In a recent scandal, consultants were alleged to be neglecting their NHS patients and doing private surgery during their contracted NHS time (Yates 1995). The author blamed private medicine, but this is typical behaviour for senior officials in a large bureaucracy where accountability, and the stimulus of competition and redundancy, have been removed. Private medicine is the solution, not the problem.

Nevertheless, the NHS generally provides reasonable care. In the curative sector the caring, enthusiasm and altruism of many health care workers maintain standards. The work is interesting, and seeing ill patients recover and be grateful encourages high standards. Unfortunately screening is different. It is repetitive and boring, with little intrinsic reward, and patients are not seen to recover and are often ungrateful. Without the incentives of competition standards inevitably fall. When the charismatic leaders who get things started move on, programmes risk degenerating into inefficient overpriced services run mainly for the benefit of disgruntled providers. It is not surprising that the press regularly exposes screening scandals, nor that the success of screening projects is rarely continued when a programme goes national.

Direct comparisons of private and public health care systems are difficult to interpret. Comparisons between countries are not very revealing since most comparable countries provide similar proportions of health care publicly. Even the United States government provides similar health expenditure to the UK government; the difference is in private provision. Such differences as do occur are confounded by other factors such as different overall wealth, ethnic mix and methods of data collection. Nevertheless some comparisons are revealing. For years child immunisation rates in the NHS-led UK have lagged behind those in the private-health-care-dominated US. Similarly overall rates of detection and treatment of hypertension have been higher in the US (JNCDETHBP 1993) than in the UK (Smith *et al* 1990). In one study American women were more likely than Canadian or German women to have undergone BP checks, Pap smears, breast examinations and mammograms in the previous year (Donelan *et al* 1996). Rates of detection and treatment of hyper-cholesterolaemia are also much higher in the United States. Since 1970 death rates from cardiovascular disease have fallen much more steeply in the US than in the UK, plausibly related to better screening and prevention.

Comparisons within countries also have problems. They rarely compare like with like and tend to be limited in the outcomes reported. When measured on the objectives the planners set themselves, planned programmes often do better than market systems in the short term. The market appears to do worse because it is responding to more diverse pressures, and long-term outcomes are rarely reported. The objectivity of publicly funded researchers is sometimes also in doubt. Nevertheless there have been some comparisons.

Comparisons Between Public and Private Health Care

Careful comparisons of public and private residential child care, taking into account possible differences in case mix, have generally concluded that the private and voluntary sectors are more efficient than the public sector (Knapp 1986), despite the latter receiving considerable invisible voluntary sector support. Similar conclusions have been drawn for residential care of the elderly (Judge 1986), although the level of care in private homes is at least as good as that in state-run ones (Barron 1996). Comparisons of dental care generally show that private provision is more efficient (Bentley *et al* 1984, Sintonen 1986), and reports showing the converse have tended to use very crude measures of output (Doherty *et al* 1980). The efficiency of private dental care is all the more impressive since private dentists practice to a higher standard, and are more likely to involve patients in treatment decisions than public ones (Forss and Widstrom 1996).

The introduction of fundholding into some general practices in the UK was a limited experiment in increasing incentives by giving doctors more control over their budgets. Fundholding practices appeared to have better relationships with hospitals, made savings on drugs budgets, and developed more practice-based services (Audit Commission 1996) although they did not implement more clinical effectiveness initiatives, do more day case surgery, or undertake health needs assessments (Stewart-Brown *et al* 1996). On one interpretation they responded to patients rather than to planners.

Although some authors criticise alleged low rates of screening in private practice in the United States, there is little objective difference in health promotion activities between health maintenance organisations (HMOs) and fee-for-service practices (Abelson and Lomas 1990). Such differences as occur (Bernstein *et al* 1991) are typically in programmes such as Pap smear, mammography, breast physical examination, digital rectal examination, and blood stool test whose cost/benefit ratio is disputed, making it hard to argue that fee-for-service patients are getting a worse service. The screening uptake rates reported in some private programmes, for example 99 per cent of patients having their blood pressure recorded, 51 per cent having a faecal occult blood screening for colon cancer (Frame *et al* 1984), would put many government screening programmes to shame. Screening performance was unrelated to payment mechanism in one comparison of 11 medical systems (Nutting *et al* 1982).

Many government screening programmes achieve very low uptake. For example the UK cervical cytology programme had low uptake until incentive payments for doctors were introduced (Health Departments of Great Britain 1989). The Canadian government-funded Pap smear screening programmes often only achieved 60 per cent uptake in the late 1980s and included a high rate of over-testing (Cohen *et al* 1992). In the UK optometrists only measure intra-ocular pressure in about half of consultations, and only measure visual fields in one in eight (Crick and Tuck 1995). The effect of the sight-test fee on glaucoma detection is unresolved (Laidlaw *et al* 1994). There may also be benefits from integrating public health programmes into the private fee-for-service health care system (Leff *et al* 1977). Removing economic barriers rarely leads to significant increases in screening (Lantz *et al* 1997) and many patients from ethnic minorities prefer being examined by 'their own' or a private physician (Williams *et al* 1997).

There have also been comparisons from other countries. In an Italian study there was better test performance from ultrasound screening for Down's syndrome in private practice than in the corresponding government clinic (Brambati *et al* 1995). In Austria private physicians are more likely to perform breast screening by palpation (Gredler and Gerstner 1987), and in Sweden a privately run, albeit publicly financed, primary health care provider delivered similar quality of care at lower cost than the publicly run services (Hansagi *et al* 1993).

A good area for comparison between private and public screening is child vaccination rates since almost everyone agrees that these should be as high as possible. Some public health physicians have suggested that private practice is inferior in this area, with a report of full immunisation rates of only 79 per cent at three months, falling to 61 per cent by two years (Bordley *et al* 1996). However, no comparison group was provided, and public paediatric clinics have reported much lower rates of 67 per cent at three months and 25 per cent at two years (Farizo *et al* 1992). The difference cannot be attributed to poor attendance by indigent parents. One study of a public clinic included only children who had attended well-child visits (an average of six such visits per child) and still reported only 73 per cent full vaccination at two years (McConnachie and Roghmann 1992). In another study missed opportunities for vaccination were more common in public than private clinics (Szilagyi *et al* 1993), resulting in higher immunisation rates among private practice patients (Szilagyi *et al* 1994). All is not perfect in private practice and in some states immunisation rates are well below target, although similar to public practice (Simpson *et al* 1997). Nevertheless, even when high rates of vaccination are achieved in public clinics, the authors often admit that these resulted from a specific initiative (Brown *et al* 1993).

It is not possible to conclude from these comparisons whether the private sector is more or less efficient than the state in providing screening. However, there is insufficient evidence to argue that the state is more efficient.

The Effect On Consumers

Government provision of health care has harmful effects on the general public. It encourages both ignorance and a complaining mentality. There is no need to complain about poor service when the market is working well, e.g. in a restaurant or supermarket. You simply go elsewhere next time, so that restaurants and supermarkets with poor service rapidly go out of business. With a near monopoly provider like the NHS it is difficult to go elsewhere, and patients either accept poor service or complain. Before long complaining becomes institutionalised both by the customers (Davies 1996), and by the providers who create patient complaints officers, complaints departments, 'patient charters' and ombudsmen, to deal with them.

Government provision also encourages ignorance. Private patients want to know what is done to them and private doctors want to keep their custom, so that gradually the whole community becomes better educated in health care. Those who are interested learn what works and what does not. The remainder either follow their lead, or learn where to go for independent advice. Everyone becomes both more demanding of good health care and more resistant to bad health propaganda. Public patients in contrast are supplicants to the doctor. They are reluctant to ask questions because they might upset their doctor, and he certainly doesn't volunteer information. Before long the community is so ignorant that providers can argue that people are not qualified to judge what they want for themselves (Orme 1996).

It is occasionally argued that state provision is 'easier' for individual consumers who can leave the decisions to experts, and spend their intellectual resources on something else. It may even reduce anxiety if charging separately for every item makes people worry about the little costs building up. In practice the private sector will offer screening packages just like the state. People who wish to decide individually about each test are free to do so, but those with better things to do with their time than worry about their health when well, simply request the 'usual' screening tests for people of their age, sex and status. The difference is that in a private system there will be a range of packages, with their contents influenced by many individual decisions.

State-Funded Prenatal Diagnosis

Inefficiency is not the only problem with state-funded screening. If the screening programme involves abortion it discriminates against the living handicapped. The problem arises because the state cannot afford to fund all possible prenatal screening, and even if it could, society would not tolerate paying for it all, so it has to draw a line over what it will fund. In the UK the NHS does not fund screening for toxoplasmosis or sex selection, decisions are being made now about cystic fibrosis and fragile X, and it is unlikely to fund screening for homosexuality, if the putative gene were identified. Such decisions cannot be made on some non-discriminatory calculation of whether the screening does more good than harm overall (Thornton and Lilford 1995), since they would require interpersonal utility comparisons that are impossible in a controversial area like abortion.

State providers could wait and see what screening programmes develop in the private market and provide only these (Thornton 1994), or give people vouchers for screening tests and let individuals decide which tests they want or whether they prefer a cash alternative (Lilford and Thornton 1996). In practice they do neither and instead provide screening arbitrarily, on the basis that some handicaps justify abortion. The short-term side-effects of this are unpleasant, with living people with handicaps for which screening is offered feeling justifiably that society does not value them, and parents of such babies feeling social pressure to have an abortion. The long-term risks of such programmes are even more serious. They put politicians on a slippery slope to funding screening for minor abnormalities. The history of eugenics does not inspire confidence that the state may not one day argue that, say, homosexuality, short stature, blue eyes or personality disorder should not be screened for (Gould 1983). If the state can draw a line at one point now there are few safeguards that it will not draw it at another point in future.

Some people find it difficult to understand why NHS screening, with the intention of aborting abnormal pregnancies, is discriminatory. This is because they only consider programmes such as those for Down's syndrome and spina bifida, for which there is no strong, articulate community of affected individuals to complain about what is going on. The recent identification of a gene mutation causing deafness (Kelsell *et al* 1997, Reardon 1998) is a better example. If the NHS offered screening for such a gene, members of the deaf community, who regard themselves as different, but in no way inferior to the hearing community, would rightly be outraged. They would be justified in opposing such NHS screening. However, unless they were opposed to abortion in general, they could not consistently oppose private individuals getting their pregnancies tested for such a gene.

None of these problems affect private testing. Individuals discriminate all the time in ways that it would be intolerable for the state to do. For example, they choose their partners on the basis of skin colour, sexual orientation, height, weight, intelligence, and physical attributes. Similarly, it is acceptable for individuals to discriminate in the children they bear on the basis of physical and mental attributes, but unacceptable for the state to do the same. Private testing programmes do not need to make any overall cost/benefit calculation. They are justified solely by their ability to increase parental choice. Parents acting individually rather than doctors acting for society, decide what abnormality is severe enough to justify screening. Even if individual parents occasionally make bad decisions, they will never all make unjust decisions on, for example, racial grounds or for trivial handicap. There is no need for society as a whole to make any decision about what abnormality is severe enough to justify screening, and therefore no risk of eugenic screening.

Summary

Private screening is more efficient and responsive to people's wants than public provision, and will often result in more testing overall. If it results in less, there must be less demand at the market price. The need to find out if a test is worth paying for forces patients to keep informed, and the stimulus of competition forces doctors to tell them what they are doing, and raises private screening standards. In contrast public programmes tend to degenerate and encourage ignorance and a complaining mentality among patients. There are special harms from public prenatal screening. It unjustly discriminates against the handicapped, and is at risk of degenerating into a eugenic programme. Health screening should be left to the private sector, unless there is a clear justification otherwise.

3

Which Programmes Should Be Provided by the State?

IN this chapter I apply the arguments from chapter two to the major screening programmes, and ask which the NHS should provide. Programmes are discussed in three sections, those directed at healthy adults, at children, and at pregnant women.

1. *Programmes Directed At Healthy Adults*

Hypertension Screening

Current status: universal adult screening offered by the NHS
Adults with high blood pressure are rarely aware of this, but they have an increased risk of strokes and heart attacks. Drug treatment prevents both diseases, but has side-effects such as reduced sexual potency or a general feeling of ill health, and some people find taking pills regularly irksome. There may even be psychological harms simply from being labelled hypertensive (Haynes *et al* 1978, Johnstone *et al* 1984). The benefits depend on the level of blood pressure, but overall many hundreds of people need to be treated to prevent one stroke and some individuals may judge this as not worthwhile, so the overall cost/benefit ratio is disputed. For men aged 45-50 the cost per life-year gained has been estimated at between £7,000 to £20,000 (Wonderling *et al* 1996), although some earlier estimates had put the figure much higher (Stenson and Weinstein 1977). Many people would prefer to spend that sort of money on other things, and since many well informed people decline even free testing, it is a want not a need. Screening has no significant externalities and is not mandated by the 'rule of rescue'.

Recommendation: the NHS should stop offering hypertension screening to healthy adults.

Cholesterol Screening

Current status: not universally offered by the NHS, widespread opportunistic screening

Like high blood pressure, raised levels of cholesterol and other types of fat in the blood increase the risk of heart attack and stroke, and can be diagnosed by a blood test. Drug treatment and a low fat diet reduces mortality, although many people find the diet unpalatable, and some people even believe that low cholesterol makes people miserable and increases suicide deaths. The degree of benefit depends on the level of raised cholesterol and, depending on the level at which treatment is started, many people need to be treated to prevent one death, so it is expensive. Much of the debate about cholesterol screening derives from controversy over whether the acknowledged benefits are worth the cost (Freemantle *et al* 1997, Muldoon and Criqui 1997, letters 1997). Estimates of the cost per life-year gained range from £48 to £130,000, with a reasonable average estimate of £7,400 (Wakeham and Leach 1997). Many people would prefer to spend that sort of money on other things. Private companies offer cholesterol screening at between £15 and £50 per test, depending on the level of subsidy. Cholesterol screening has no significant externalities, so the arguments for the NHS not getting involved are the same as those for hypertension screening.

Recommendation: the NHS should not screen for hyper-cholesterolaemia.

Screening Packages For Cardiovascular Risk

Current status: not universally offered by the NHS, widespread opportunistic screening

Many people have wondered whether screening for a package of heart disease risk factors, typically blood pressure, weight and cholesterol, and smoking and alcohol consumption, might be worthwhile. This reduces risk factors for heart attacks by about 12 per cent (ICRF OXCHECK Study Group 1995, Family Heart Study Group 1994), so that, if translated into reduced mortality, the cost would be about £8,000 per life-year gained. This figure is subject to considerable uncertainties and estimates range from

£1,000 to £144,000 depending on age and sex (Wonderling *et al* 1996). It is hardly surprising that people disagree about whether it is worthwhile. Enthusiasts for private screening argue that individuals screened by the NHS are less likely to comply with the advice than those who requested screening privately. Cynics also question whether the efficiency of publicly funded programmes could be maintained long term in the NHS. Like hypertension and cholesterol screening separately, many people would prefer to spend this sort of money elsewhere, the market cost is £160 (BUPA), and only a tiny percentage of people pay this. Few people even pay the subsidised charity cost of £55 (Marie Stopes). It is a want rather than a need.

Recommendation: the NHS should not screen adults for cardiovascular risk.

Cervical Cancer

Current status: universal screening offered by the NHS
This caused 1,333 deaths in 1995 in England and Wales (ONS 1996). Most cases pass through a pre-cancerous stage in which abnormal cells can be identified and destroyed. The test for pre-cancer, the Pap, or smear test, involves a vaginal examination, and is offered to women every three years in the NHS. If abnormal cells are found they can be cut away with a knife or laser. Occasionally women who have completed their family choose to undergo hysterectomy. Most experts believe this reduces deaths from cervical cancer (Hakama *et al* 1985) but the side-effects are important, there are many false positives, and much pre-cancer regresses spontaneously. Many women never destined to get cancer are made anxious, and some have unnecessary operations. Since the risk of cervical cancer increases with sexual promiscuity, abnormal smear results can provoke marital discord. Some women regard the programme as not worthwhile, either because they particularly dislike vaginal examinations, or because they believe themselves to be at low risk.

The cost per life-year gained has been estimated at around £9,000 (Wakeham and Leach 1997), the market cost is around £50 per test (BUPA) and the subsidised charitable cost around half that (Marie Stopes). The cost/benefit ratio is disputed. A substantial minority of women avoids even free cervical testing, and many would not pay for it, if given the choice. It is a want not a need and there are no externalities. Some will argue that cervical cancer is a disease of poverty, and that removing free screening from poor people will increase their deprivation. However, poor women are low attendees, even for free cervical cytology screening. They can be persuaded to undergo testing if it is offered when they come for other reasons, but this hardly indicates real demand. Unless doctors know the priorities of poor women better then the women themselves, we must assume that the programme is not cost/beneficial to such women. If so, providing it free does not alleviate poverty even if it reduces their mortality.

If the NHS stopped supplying it to healthy adult women, the range of private providers would expand, and those women who want it enough to pay for it would get it. Providers would know which social groups were most at risk and have an incentive to direct some of their advertising accordingly. If low-cost private screening programmes succeeded that would indicate that the programme was cost/beneficial to at least some relatively poor women. If they did not that would confirm that poor women have other priorities. Those middle-class people who felt strongly that such women were being deprived would still be free to fund low-cost or free cervical screening charities (see chapter 4).

Recommendation: the NHS should stop screening for cervical cancer.

Breast Cancer

Current status: screening offered by the NHS to all women age 50 to 64

Nearly one in ten UK women develop breast cancer during their lifetime. The best screening test is an X-ray of the breast, or mammogram, which in the NHS is repeated every three years. Suspicious areas are biopsied, either by means of a small operation or with a fine needle, and, if cancer is diagnosed, the lump or the whole breast is removed. This reduces breast cancer mortality in older women (Cuckle 1991), although there is some doubt whether it is equally effective in younger women. About 75 per cent of women under 65 take up the offer of a free test but many older women dislike the procedure, which they find both undignified and uncomfortable, and the radiation dose, albeit low, concerns some people. One in 20 women require recall for further mammogram and one in a hundred require biopsy of which one in eight turn out to be cancerous (Wald 1994). The estimated cost per life-year gained is similar to cervical cytology at £8,500 (Wakeham and Leach 1997). The market cost is £85 per test (BUPA) and the cost/benefit ratio is disputed because of the false positives, anxiety, cosmetic damage from unnecessary surgery and radiation risk. Many women decline even free screening, and even more would choose not to pay for it. It is a want not a need.

The argument that free screening alleviates poverty has even less force than with cervical screening, because breast cancer is more common among the middle classes. Perhaps that is why NHS breast screening services tend to be better resourced than cervical ones! A recent campaign to extend routine mammography invitations to women over 64 (Sutton 1997) demonstrates the coercion implicit in NHS screening. Although women over this age can already be screened free on request, less than two per cent of such women avail themselves of this facility.

Recommendation: the NHS should stop screening for breast cancer.

Bowel Cancer

Current status: not universally offered by the NHS, widespread opportunistic screening

This causes over 15,000 deaths annually in England and Wales (ONS 1996). Screening involves testing the stool for blood, and, if positive, inserting a tube into the anus (colonoscopy) to look for polyps, some of which are pre-cancerous. This is probably effective but there are many false positives, and occasional serious complications from colonoscopy. Many people find collecting and testing their stool distasteful. The risk/benefit ratio varies with age and family history (Dunlop and Campbell 1997) and, because of false positives, is disputed. The American Cancer Society recommends annual tests for everyone aged over 50, although the

United States government does not pay for this. Opinion leaders in the NHS have decided that it is not overall worthwhile. There are no externalities, so the NHS is correct to not screen for it, and patients can decide for themselves.

Recommendation: the NHS should not screen for bowel cancer.

Ovarian Cancer

Current status: not offered by the NHS

This causes nearly 4,000 deaths annually in England and Wales (ONS 1996) and can be screened for by a blood test or a vaginal ultrasound examination. Neither is suitable for pre-menopausal women because of false positives but all older women are eligible. If either test is positive, removing the ovary both confirms the cancer and hopefully cures it. This probably prevents some deaths, but many women will undergo unnecessary surgery and many older women dislike vaginal examinations, so the cost/benefit ratio is disputed. Some people pay for it privately so it must be worthwhile to them, but most people regard it as not worth the side-effects. So far opinion leaders in the NHS have decided that it is not worthwhile and it is not currently offered. Since there are no externalities this is correct and adult women can decide for themselves.

Recommendation: the NHS should not screen for ovarian cancer.

Prostate Cancer

Current status: not offered by the NHS

This is the third leading cause of cancer deaths in men in England and Wales with nearly 9,000 deaths annually (ONS 1996). Although the early asymptomatic stage may be curable with surgery, the screening blood test for prostate specific antigen is relatively non-specific. Many patients have an abnormal result without cancer, or with only a very early slow growing tumour, which would not cause trouble within their lifetime. This cannot always be predicted, so some men undergo treatment unnecessarily. Since the surgery often causes impotence and incontinence, and may have little effect on overall survival, most expert groups have concluded that screening is not cost/beneficial (USPSTF

1996, NHS CRD 1997). However, individuals who place a relatively high value on life, compared with sexual function, may judge things differently (Krahn *et al* 1994). It is included in BUPA's full health screening package and Marie Stopes offers it at a subsidised rate of £25. Whether this enthusiasm will persist, as the side-effects and doubts about effectiveness are more widely reported, will be revealed by the future success of such private programmes. For the moment it is worthwhile for some, but not for others, and NHS opinion leaders have decided not to provide it. It is a want not a need and offering it free to poor people will not alleviate poverty. There are no beneficial externalities, so this decision is correct.

Recommendation: the NHS should not screen for prostate cancer.

Tests for Genetic Diseases

Current status: not universally offered by the NHS
The mutations responsible for many genetic diseases have been already identified, or soon will be. When this is done they can be screened for by a simple blood test or mouth wash. The two best established are sickle cell disease and cystic fibrosis. At present neither of these diseases are curable and treatment is directed at mitigating symptoms, so there is little direct benefit to affected individuals from screening. If carrying an abnormal gene increases illness or shortens life expectancy there may even be a harm in that health and life insurance will be more difficult to obtain. The main benefit comes to healthy carriers of the genes who can avoid having affected children either by choosing their partner carefully or by selective abortion. People's views differ so widely that it is impossible to make an overall cost/benefit calculation. There are no externalities and this is not a public good.

Recommendation: the NHS should not offer adult screening for genetic diseases.

Vision Screening

Current status: adult screening not universally offered by the NHS
Most adult vision problems, such as refractive disorders and

cataract, can be treated when vision becomes impaired. An exception is chronic glaucoma where treatment before symptoms develop may prevent blindness. Screening is done by optometrists checking the intra-ocular pressure, or the visual fields. Some people argue that treatment is not very effective, many people are treated unnecessarily (Wormald *et al* 1997), and it is diverting resources from curative eye services (Griffiths 1997). A fall in NHS screening followed the introduction of the fee, presumably indicating that some people prefer to spend their money on something else (Laidlaw *et al* 1994). There are no externalities.

Recommendation: the NHS should not screen for adult vision problems.

Tuberculosis

Current status: selective screening of high risk groups is offered by the NHS

Sputum examination, chest X-ray and skin tests for tuberculosis are long established, and effective drug treatment is available. The main harm is radiation from the X-rays. Since TB is now rare in the general population, screening is usually focused on high-risk groups, such as health workers and the homeless. It may not even be worthwhile to the homeless. They don't spend their disposable income on it, and frequently decline even free screening, presumably because they have other priorities. Nevertheless, it is reasonable for the state to offer it to them. Many are mentally disabled in one way or another, so that the state is justified in overriding their preferences, and there is a beneficial externality from reducing transmission of TB to third parties.

Recommendation: selective NHS screening for TB in high risk groups should continue.

Sexually Transmitted Diseases Including HIV/AIDS

Current status: universal contact tracing (screening) offered by NHS

Syphilis and HIV/AIDS can be screened for by a blood test, while other sexually transmitted infections can be detected by genital examination. General population screening would be unpopular because people would be upset by the implied moral censure of receiving an invitation. Screening the sexual contacts of people with a sexually transmitted disease is effective, and benefits not only those who turn out to be affected but their future sexual contacts. Some people might pay privately for contact tracing but others would not. However, the beneficial externality justifies state provision, or at least state subsidy of private providers. Similarly, screening high-risk groups such as sex workers is effective, but the cost/benefit ratio will be disputed because some will argue that it encourages immoral behaviour. Nevertheless, the beneficial externality of reducing transmission to third parties might justify it.

Recommendation: NHS contact tracing for sexually transmitted infections should continue.

Adult Screening Summary

The state should not provide screening for adults unless there is either a beneficial externality, or a programme of undoubted cost/benefit helps the poor. Wrong decisions have been made in the past because the role of the state in providing health care has not been properly defined. There is no fundamental difference between the programmes provided by the NHS (hypertension, cervical cytology and mammography for women aged 50-64) and many of those not currently offered (cholesterol, faecal occult blood, ovarian cancer screening, and mammography for women aged under 50 or over 64). They are all effective, but their cost/benefit ratios are disputed. We know this because many prudent people decline them even when they are free, and even more prudent people don't bother to spend their own money on them. None of them are public goods or have significant beneficial externalities. The state should not provide them. Effective programmes directed at the mentally handicapped, or with beneficial externalities, such as tuberculosis screening for the homeless, and sexually transmitted disease contact tracing, should continue.

If the NHS stops hypertension, cervical cytology and mammography screening, and fails to introduce screening for bowel and ovarian cancer and for hyper-cholesterolaemia, vested interests will start shroud-waving. People with serious disease who had not bothered to get themselves screened might appear in the media, claiming that they did not know about it, or had not been able to afford it. It would be argued that the state had a duty to do some thing about such people. Similarly, if people felt deprived by not having screening, they would demand it from their GP. What action would the rule of rescue mandate?

The government should explain that adults should look after their own preventive health care. The worth of screening depends on an individual's preferences, and it should be up to individuals to decide if they want to pay for it. The rule of rescue would be satisfied if the state provided responsive testing for those who demand it. This already happens with cholesterol testing and screening for bowel and ovarian cancer, and for women outside the present age range for mammography invitations. Few people take up such tests without heavy NHS propaganda.

2. *Programmes Directed at Children*

Guthrie Screening

Current status: universal screening by the NHS

Phenyl-ketonuria is a rare genetic condition that affects one in 20,000 births. Affected babies appear normal at birth but develop progressive brain damage in early childhood. Screening involves measuring phenylalanine levels in a blood spot on filter paper taken 3-5 days after delivery, the Guthrie test. Affected children are given a phenylalanine free diet which, while somewhat inconvenient, is effective. Significant handicap from phenyl-ketonuria is now rare. Guthrie testing is cheap, has no important side-effects, and the cost/benefit ratio is highly favourable (Torrance and Zipursky 1984). Even if it were not provided free, all prudent parents would pay for it. However, the disadvantage of leaving it to parents to arrange privately would be that some imprudent ones would fail to do so and their children would be avoidably damaged. Given the benefits, and minimal harm, such parents would not be acting in the best interests of their child. State coercion is justified to help the deprived, in this case the children of ignorant, lazy or feckless parents. If the state did not provide it, the presence of avoidably handicapped children in society would mandate action according to the rule of rescue.

Recommendation: NHS screening should continue

New-born Thyroid Screening

Current status: universal screening by the NHS

Genetic hypothyroidism affects one in 4,000 births. Without treatment infants become severely mentally handicapped. The old fashioned name was cretinism. All newborn babies can be tested by a blood spot on filter paper, usually the same one as used for the Guthrie test. Affected infants are given thyroid hormone, and cretinism is now rare, largely due to effective screening. Few doubt that this is cost/ beneficial (Epstein *et al* 1981). Although occasional false positives cause anxiety (Tymstra 1986), the same arguments apply as for Guthrie testing.

Recommendation: NHS screening should continue

Cystic Fibrosis

Current status: not universally offered by the NHS

This is a serious genetic disease affecting one in 2,000 births. A simple test on the Guthrie blood spot permits diagnosis before it would have presented naturally. Until recently, the benefit was to permit parents to make reproductive choices such as prenatal diagnosis and abortion, and people disagreed as to whether it was worthwhile. However, with modern treatment, early diagnosis may improve outcome for the child itself (Wisconsin Cystic Fibrosis Neonatal Screening Group 1997), and, if this is confirmed, NHS screening may in future be justified.

Recommendation: at present the NHS should not screen for cystic fibrosis.

Tandem Mass Spectrometry

Current status: not universally offered by NHS

There are about 17 other congenital metabolic diseases which can be screened for in the newborn period, using the Guthrie blood spots and a special laboratory test known as tandem mass spectrometry (Pollitt 1997). The benefit of screening for the treatable ones is clear, but for untreatable diseases screening simply prolongs the period over which parents know their child is ill. In these latter cases the benefit lies in permitting parents to not have more children, or to undergo prenatal diagnosis and selective abortion, and it is therefore disputed. NHS screening is only justified for the former.

Recommendation: the NHS should screen by tandem mass spectrometry only for treatable diseases.

The New-born Physical Examination

Current status: universal screening by NHS
In most developed countries all newborn babies are examined soon after birth for congenital defects. These include obvious abnormalities which few parents would miss, such as limb defects and birth marks, subtle ones which parents may not detect immediately, such as Down's syndrome and cleft palate, and those which can only be detected by a trained person, such as heart murmurs and dislocation of the hip. The effectiveness is uncertain. Parents would pick up most treatable disease in time, screening often detects trivial or non-existent disease that alarms parents, and a negative examination may falsely reassure parents. The most important abnormality detected by this screen is congenital dislocation of the hip. This is a preventable cause of lameness, which particularly affects girls. Without screening it would not be detected until the child started walking and early diagnosis may improve prognosis. Although screening by clinical or ultrasound examination is probably effective, some children get unnecessary treatment, so its overall cost/benefit is disputed. If it were not already current practice there would be no need for the state to introduce it. However, all mothers now expect it and would demand it if the NHS dropped it. Cases would soon appear where it was alleged that lack of it had caused avoidable handicap, so it would be mandated by the rule of rescue.

Recommendation: the NHS new-born examination should continue.

Immunisation Status

Current status: universal screening by the NHS
This is a particularly effective screening programme. Immunisation prevents diphtheria, tetanus, whooping cough, measles, rubella and polio. By simply checking a child's health record, those who have not received the recommended doses can have the deficiencies remedied. Although there may be serious side-effects from some immunisations such as whooping cough, which some parents prefer their children to avoid, hardly anyone disputes that most programmes are cost/ beneficial. NHS screening helps the children of the poor who might otherwise tend to miss out.

Recommendation: NHS screening of children for immunisation status should continue.

Vision Screening

Current status: universal screening by the NHS
Child vision screening involves full sight-testing, because children and parents can be unaware of mild visual impairment. The main benefit results from treatment of mild amblyopia (squint) which, it is believed, can progress if untreated to blindness in the affected eye. Screening is regarded as effective in North America (USPSTF 1996) but the evidence is not conclusive and a recent UK review concluded that the evidence was insufficient for providers to continue offering it (Snowdon and Stewart-Brown 1997). The problem is that the natural history of untreated mild amblyopia is uncertain and the treatments may often be unnecessary or ineffective. Nevertheless it would be difficult to withdraw such a well-established NHS programme without provoking shroud-waving which it would be difficult to ignore.
Recommendation: NHS vision screening of children should continue

3. *Pregnancy Screening Programmes*

Pregnant women are often tested to prevent disease in the baby. Fortunately mothers can usually be relied on to act in their baby's best interest and there is only a limited role for the state in ensuring that fetuses are not avoidably harmed by mothers making idiosyncratic choices, or dealing with externalities.

Screening for untreatable fetal disease is a special case, because of abortion. It can have a dramatic impact. Congenital diseases often cause many years of ill health so that, if an abnormal pregnancy is aborted and the parents have another healthy child who would otherwise have never been conceived, considerable suffering is avoided. Even allowing for the anxiety of testing, the unpleasantness of abortion, and the occasional miscarriage of a normal baby, many people feel that the gains outweigh the side-effects. There may also be economic gains to the rest of society.

The problem is that abortion is unacceptable to many people. In a recent UK survey only 66 per cent of people approved of abortion when the child was likely to be born mentally or physically handicapped, and one in five actively disapproved of abortion for this reason (Wise 1997). There are nearly 2,000 such abortions in England and Wales each year (ONS 1996), most of which are the direct result of NHS screening. Although no one is forced to undergo either testing or abortion and medical staff, at least in theory, try to avoid coercion, many women claim to feel pressurised to undergo testing and to act on the result. Many studies have shown how prenatal clinic staff are biased in the way they inform parents about the tests. They often refer to a handicap risk of one in 200 as 'high', while calling a one in 100 risk of miscarriage 'low'. Even if they are scrupulously non-directive, parents may assume that the offer of testing itself carries medical endorsement. Some people argue that it is impossible to be unbiased (Clarke 1991). Nevertheless, many pregnancy screening programmes for treatable and untreatable disease are available. Some are funded by the state and described below.

The Prenatal Care Package

Current status: pregnancy screening for hypertension, diabetes, malpresentation, fetal growth restriction and many other disorders, is widely offered by the NHS.

Repeated clinical examinations by midwives or doctors at progressively decreasing intervals in pregnancy form the package of prenatal care. The aim is to detect such asymptomatic diseases as hypertension, early diabetes, urinary infection, malpresentations, and poor fetal growth. The system is probably effective in preventing serious disease in both mother and baby, although it is inconvenient and expensive, and some women might prefer to forego it. If only the mother's health were involved it would be better provided privately, but NHS provision may be justified to protect unborn children.

Recommendation: the NHS should continue to provide a package of effective prenatal care.

Rubella

Current status: universal screening by the NHS
Rubella (German measles) is a relatively mild viral infection that usually affects young children. Adults rarely suffer serious consequences, but in pregnancy the infection may cause deafness, congenital heart disease, and brain damage to the baby. Before immunisation was offered 100 to 200 infants were damaged this way in the UK each year. Although children are now immunised at school, some manage to miss it and can be identified by testing in pregnancy. Although too late to help their present pregnancy, those that are non-immune can be offered immunisation when the baby is born. This protects subsequent babies and is cheap and non-controversial. Prudent parents would all want testing, but some lazy or ignorant ones might not bother. State screening will prevent serious damage to their children, and is justified in the child's interest. If it were not provided, it would soon be mandated by the rule of rescue.

Recommendation: NHS prenatal screening for rubella non immunity should continue.

Rhesus Disease

Current status: universal screening by the NHS
This is highly effective. One in ten mothers are blood group rhesus negative and at risk of developing an antibody against their baby's blood during pregnancy, which in later pregnancies may cause anaemia, jaundice or brain damage after delivery. Rhesus disease used to kill nearly 1,000 babies each year in the UK, but now all pregnant women have their blood group checked and those at risk have a preventive injection after delivery. The process needs repeating in subsequent pregnancies but is so effective that rhesus disease is now almost entirely confined to babies of women who missed the preventive dose. The screening does not even seem to

cause anxiety because there is no stigma attached to being rhesus negative and the treatment is almost guaranteed to work. The only possible side-effect is transmission of infection, because the preventative injection is sometimes extracted from human blood. With the development of genetically engineered treatment this risk will disappear. For the same reason a few members of fundamentalist religious groups (e.g. Jehovah's Witnesses) refuse it. Nevertheless the overall benefit is not disputed, the cost per life-year saved is tiny (Torrance and Zipursky 1984) and all prudent parents would pay for it if they had to. The state should provide it for the same reason as rubella non-immunity screening.

Recommendation: NHS prenatal screening for blood group and rhesus antibodies should continue.

Syphilis

Current status: universal screening by the NHS

This used to be a major cause of miscarriage, stillbirth and neonatal handicap, but with screening and treatment it now affects only 2-5/10,000 pregnancies. Currently all pregnant women undergo a blood test and those with syphilis are treated and advised to inform their sexual contacts. Although many people are tested for each new treatable case, the test and treatment are so cheap that the overall cost is still low. Syphilis rates might increase in future if AIDS enters the heterosexual population to a significant extent, and there are beneficial externalities from treating the rare cases of syphilis that are identified. The programme appears to be acceptable to the general population, although many people are probably unaware that it is going on. Since the beneficiaries of treatment include children, it remains justified for the state to continue screening.

Recommendation: NHS prenatal screening for syphilis should continue.

HIV/AIDS

Current status: screening not universally offered by the NHS

Screening for maternal HIV infection by a blood test is not generally offered in the UK, partly because, until recently, the only treatment option was abortion. However, new drug treatments may reduce the risk of HIV transmission to the child, so there is now pressure for the NHS to offer testing to all pregnant women. Opponents argue that HIV infection is so rare in most social groups that the anxiety caused and opportunity costs foregone outweigh the gains. People opposed to abortion object because many HIV positive women still choose abortion rather than treatment. Enthusiasts counter that there will be beneficial externalities if HIV positive people alter their sexual behaviour. The enthusiasts are correct in principle. State screening protects the disadvantaged and reduces adverse externalities. Whether it is worth the opportunity costs depends on the risk of HIV/AIDS in any particular community.

Recommendation: NHS screening for HIV may be justified if the population risk is sufficiently high.

Down's Syndrome

Current status: not universally offered by the NHS, screening for older women widespread

Affected children are mentally and sometimes also physically handicapped, with 600 affected births per year in the UK. Screening involves asking the mother her age (the risk rises with age), testing her blood, or looking for subtle abnormalities in the baby by ultrasound examination. None of these tests can make the diagnosis for certain, but they can identify pregnancies at high risk so that parents can decide whether to undergo a diagnostic test, usually amniocentesis. A needle is passed into the womb through the mother's abdomen and about 20 mls of the amniotic fluid is withdrawn. This contains skin cells from the baby that can be tested and, if there is an extra chromosome number 21, abortion is offered. Apart from the issue of abortion, the problems are that amniocentesis carries a risk (about one per cent) of causing miscarriage of a normal baby, and the results take up to three weeks, which is an unavoidably anxious time for the parents.

Screening by blood test or ultrasound is effective and cheap (£50-£100). The net costs to the state might even be negative when the savings in caring for the handicapped births prevented are taken into account. However the cost/benefit ratio depends on how people value the anxiety of a false positive result, and how individual parents value abortion, miscarriage of a wanted pregnancy and the birth of a handicapped child. Not surprisingly, it is hotly disputed. There is no objective way to decide whether Down's screening, or any other similar screening, is cost/beneficial to society. It seems to be more of a want than a need, since relatively few of even wealthy mothers bother to buy tests, even in those areas where NHS screening is not offered. A decision to provide it free by the state is arbitrary.

State provision cannot be justified to relieve poverty. The poor do not suffer an excess Down's. In contrast they tend to have children relatively young, and may even suffer less. Free screening may result in the poor getting more testing than they want, if they accept a free test to please their doctor. This would not matter if everyone agreed that screening was worthwhile, but they do not. If the programme is harmful, people may be having it inflicted because they find it difficult to decline a free test. The externalities are also harmful. Even private testing and abortion may make the existing handicapped feel undervalued. This is a pity, but it does not justify refusing to let people pay for testing if they wish. The externality becomes important if the state gets involved. The decision to fund it can only be justified by assuming that the lives of people with Down's syndrome are of less value than those of healthy people. The rule of rescue does not mandate state screening for Down's. There is no identified handicapped person to rescue. Even if people appear in the media with Down's children arguing that their birth would have been avoided by screening, it will be difficult to argue that the state should provide that screening. To do so would require the argument that the identified person with Down's would have been better off aborted.

Recommendation: the NHS should not offer screening for Down's syndrome.

Spina Bifida

Current status: universal screening by the NHS

This is a serious abnormality, affecting one or two per 1,000 births in the UK. The spine, and sometimes also the brain, fails to develop properly and severe cases die soon after birth, whatever is done.

With treatment, mild cases may have a fairly normal life expectancy, but often require multiple operations and have problems walking and passing urine. Some are wheelchair-bound and need a permanent urinary catheter. Some also have mild mental handicap. There are two methods of screening. The first is a blood test similar to that for Down's syndrome. If it indicates a sufficiently high risk, amniocentesis can make the diagnosis. There is no prenatal treatment so, like Down's syndrome, the only option is abortion.* This blood screening is believed to be largely responsible for the considerable fall in the birth incidence of spina bifida over the last 25 years. The alternative of ultrasound examination is popular but may miss some cases, or identify other problems that may be more or less severe than spina bifida. This is a mixed blessing. Many severe abnormalities would miscarry anyway, and although parents may be glad that they were prepared for an abnormal birth, it is rare for early diagnosis to make much difference to the physical outcome. Occasionally parents choose abortion for a relatively mild abnormality detected by ultrasound.

Serum and ultrasound screening for spina bifida are both effective. However, there are no beneficial externalities, they are not public goods, or mandated by the rule of rescue. All the arguments against NHS screening for Down's syndrome apply with two minor differences. The first is that spina bifida may be slightly more common among the poor, so that some might argue that government screening helps them. It does not, for the same reasons that giving poor people other free screening programmes of disputed cost/benefit does not help them. Spina bifida screening is a want not a need. Although we help some poor people by giving them their wants, we harm others because it is not cost/beneficial to them. We can only be sure of helping them by giving the equivalent money, and letting them decide whether to spend it on screening. If we don't want to do that our motivation must be to prevent the birth of poor babies with spina bifida. Such paternalistic persuasion of the poor to undergo prenatal screening and abortion cannot be justified. The other

---

* If treatment *in utero* turns out to be successful and safe for the mother NHS screening may one day be mandated in the child's interest (Adzick *et al* 1998).

difference is that there is a small extra adverse externality. Spina bifida is preventable in many cases by vitamin supplements before conception, but, insofar as screening reduces the birth prevalence, it may weaken such efforts at primary prevention.

Recommendation: the NHS should not offer screening for spina bifida.

Cystic Fibrosis

Current status: not universally offered by the NHS

In pregnancy screening for cystic fibrosis the mother is usually tested first, and the father tested if she is a carrier. If both parents are carriers the unborn baby can be tested by amniocentesis and abortion offered if it is affected. This works, but because of concerns that it may not be cost-effective and that cystic fibrosis is not a sufficiently serious disease, the NHS does not yet offer it as a routine. The same arguments apply as for Down's and spina bifida. Less informed people tend to undergo more cystic fibrosis testing in pregnancy (Thornton *et al* 1995), and outside pregnancy many people accept cystic fibrosis testing offered immediately, but do not return on another day for the same free test (Bekker *et al* 1993). Clearly their desire to be tested is not strong. This is a reason why the poor might actually benefit from the state not providing it free. They avoid being passively coerced into accepting tests they do not really want.

Recommendation: the NHS should not offer prenatal screening for cystic fibrosis.

Ultrasound Screening

Current status: universal screening by the NHS

It is a recurring theme of this book that NHS screening with the aim of preventing disease in babies can often be justified, but that screening to permit abortion of babies with untreatable disease should be left to the private sector. Ultrasound screening may have both effects.

Nevertheless screening for structural abnormalities can usually be separated from simple obstetric scanning. It has to be done at the correct time (18-20 weeks) and requires skilled staff to deliberately take carefully orientated views of the fetus. Such high-level scanning prevents the birth of babies with major abnormalities by permitting abortion, but the cost/benefit is difficult to calculate. Some abnormalities are lethal anyway, and for many others prenatal diagnosis makes little difference to the outcome. Parents occasionally choose abortion for minor abnormalities, and occasionally mistakes are made and normal babies aborted for non-existent abnormalities. Even trivial abnormalities cause considerable parental anxiety. However, ultrasound scanning is popular with parents who like to see the baby and always hope that it will give them reassurance that everything is normal. At least 99 per cent of parents request a free scan for anatomy however much they are warned about the risks (Thornton *et al* 1995). Most women indicate that they would be willing to pay large sums for a scan if necessary (Berwick and Weinstein 1985), and those undergoing private prenatal care usually pay for ultrasound even if they decline other tests. Nevertheless the benefits in terms of the pleasure of seeing the baby and checking for obstetric problems could be achieved without searching for anatomical problems. The case against anatomical screening in time for abortion is the same as that against any other screen for untreatable abnormality. The cost/benefit calculation involves abortion and handicap and cannot and should not be made at the population level. Such scanning should be left to the private sector and not offered by the NHS.

There are many other reasons for pregnancy scanning, including checking the gestational age, counting the babies, ensuring they are alive and growing normally, and locating the placenta. This is sometimes called low-level scanning. Most of it is done in response to a clinical problem or a maternal worry, and is therefore not screening. If it turns up fetal abnormalities, they have to be dealt with as best they can. If there were evidence that such routine low-level scanning benefited the baby NHS provision might be justified, but this is not the case at present.

Recommendation: universal NHS high-level ultrasound screening of fetal anatomy at 18 to 20 weeks should stop. Low-level ultrasound scanning at other gestational ages should be limited to obstetric indications or in response to maternal demand.

Haemoglobinopathy (Sickle Cell Disease, Beta Thalassaemia)

Current status: screening of at-risk groups offered by the NHS

Sickle cell disease affects people of African origin. The severity varies, but typically children have repeated episodes of pain and, sooner or later, develop kidney or lung failure or suffer strokes. With modern treatment, the average life expectancy is about 50 years. Beta Thalassaemia, in contrast, is common around the Mediterranean and the Far East, affecting one in 400 babies in some areas. It is more severe than sickle cell disease. Without treatment, children die in early childhood, and even with treatment most die in their teens. Both diseases are inherited in a recessive pattern with children being affected if they inherit an abnormal gene from both parents.

The screening blood test for these genes is usually offered to mothers at risk, namely those whose ancestors came from Africa, the Mediterranean and the Far East. If she is a carrier, her partner is also tested and, if he is also a carrier, there is a one-in-four chance of the child being affected. An amniocentesis or chorionic villus sampling test can be done to test the baby and, if it is affected, abortion can be offered. Screening for carrier status of these conditions is effective but the cost/benefit ratio differs between individuals. With the exception of the Cypriot population of London, among whom Thalassaemia testing is popular, there is little real demand from the ethnic groups concerned. When screening has been offered to people of West Indian origin (at risk of sickle cell disease), or the Pakistani populations of Bradford, Birmingham and Leicester (at risk of Thalassaemia), uptake rates have been low. Enthusiasts have argued that this is due to ignorance of the service and provided a range of link workers and genetic counsellors to 'educate' them. As a result uptake rates have risen, although many people still decline the tests actively, or manage to avoid testing by attending for prenatal care too late. These screening programmes are at best paternalistic, and at worst racist. The fact that hardly any people from those cultures pay for such screening despite usually being well able to afford it, or even ask for it from the NHS, indicates that many of them do not regard it as cost/beneficial. The case against it is the same as that for other prenatal diagnosis of untreatable disease, with the additional objection of its racist overtones.

Recommendation: the NHS should not offer screening for haemoglobinopathy.

Tay Sach's Disease

Current status: screening not offered by the NHS

This rare genetic disease affects one in 4,000 babies among Ashkenazi Jews. There is no treatment. Affected babies develop progressive mental and motor deterioration and blindness, and die usually by five years. Screening is done by a blood test on the parents. If both are carriers, the fetus can be tested by amniocentesis or chorionic villus biopsy and abortion offered. Young single people can also be tested to avoid carriers marrying. Screening is effective and does not carry the racist overtones of haemoglobinopathy screening, since most programmes have been initiated and maintained by members of the population at risk, Ashkenazi Jews. However, all the other arguments apply, and the NHS should not screen for it.

Recommendation: the NHS should not offer screening for Tay Sach's.

Fragile X

Current status: screening not offered by the NHS.

This prenatal screening test has recently been developed. Fragile X is a genetic disease that is carried by women but mainly affects boys. It usually, although not invariably, causes severe mental handicap. Women can be tested to see if they are carriers, the fetus can be sexed, and, if male, can be tested for the gene. If a son has inherited the gene, parents can be offered abortion. NHS screening would probably be effective and has been recommended on the grounds that the costs of screening are less than the costs of caring for such children (Cuckle *et al* 1997). However, like other genetic tests, the cost/benefit is for parents to decide. One problem is that some women carriers are mildly mentally retarded and might legitimately be felt to be unable to make a fully informed decision. However, if the state provides screening it would be easy to coerce women carriers into accepting it. The spectre of the state persuading a group of mildly handicapped women to undergo testing so that they can be offered abortion of their more severely handicapped children is not attractive. It would be preferable if the decision to advise such women was left to their partners and relations and, if people feel strongly about it, to charities.

Recommendation: the NHS should not screen for fragile X.

Toxoplasmosis

Current status: screening is not offered by the NHS,
Toxoplasma gondii is a protozoa which infects cats and occasionally humans. It does not usually cause problems in adults but in pregnancy it may infect the baby causing the disease toxoplasmosis. Between ten and 60 infants are severely handicapped from this cause in the UK annually, although the exact figure is vigorously disputed. Screening involves testing all mothers at the start of pregnancy for evidence of past infection. Those without such evidence are at risk of infection in future and are tested repeatedly through the pregnancy. If they get infected, blood is taken from the fetus and, if it also has been infected, abortion or treatment with antibiotics can be offered. The problems are that the tests are difficult to interpret, so normal pregnancies may be terminated as a result of false positive results, and there is little hard evidence that the antibiotic treatment helps. The disease is so rare in the UK that the number of normal babies aborted as a side-effect of screening would be similar to the number of handicapped births prevented. It may be cost/beneficial for some, but opinion leaders in the UK have decided not to screen for it. Although that decision is arbitrary it is correct. Transmission does not occur from person to person so there are no beneficial externalities from screening.

Recommendation: the NHS should not offer screening for toxoplasmosis.

Deafness

Current status: screening is not offered by the NHS
Isolated genetic deafness affects about one in 2,000 births, and a mutation in a gene, Connexin 26, has recently been identified as causing most cases (Kelsell *et al* 1997, Reardon 1998). It would be technically possible to screen parents for this mutation and offer abortion of affected pregnancies. However, the ethical problems are

even greater than for other abortion-related screening. Even without screening, doctors involved in prenatal diagnosis have received some tricky requests. Not only have hearing parents asked for testing to abort deaf children, but deaf parents have considered testing to abort hearing children (Middleton per communication). This may seem outlandish to people with no contact with the deaf community, but for deaf people having a hearing child may be as difficult to cope with as having a deaf child is for hearing parents (Middleton *et al* 1998). Such children need outsiders to help them speak well, and often have difficulties integrating in both the deaf community of their parents and the outside, hearing world. Frequently they lose touch with their parents relatively early in life.

The medical *response* to such parental requests is not the subject of this book. Here I consider whether the NHS should *initiate* such requests by offering free prenatal gene screening. If it did, members of the deaf community would be outraged. They do not accept the implication of NHS screening that they are in some way inferior to hearing people, and they would also be fearful that their whole community might eventually cease to exist. They would be completely justified in opposing such NHS screening. Screening for deafness is not a public good, there are no beneficial externalities, it does not help the poor, and the rule of rescue is not involved.

Recommendation: the NHS should not offer screening for deafness.

Summary For Prenatal Screening

The NHS may be justified in screening to prevent disease in the baby on the grounds that babies who cannot look after themselves would otherwise be at risk of damage from the neglect of feckless parents. Similarly government screening for some infectious diseases may be justified because of the externalities. However NHS provision of prenatal screening for the abortion of babies with untreatable disease is not justified. It does not provide an otherwise unobtainable public good, and is not mandated by the rule of rescue. It probably does not help the poor—being given the equivalent money would help them more—and any beneficial effect on poverty does not justify the harm. It causes moral hazard, discriminates against the handicapped more than private screening, and its arbitrary nature makes it potentially eugenic. Existing state-funded prenatal screening programmes for congenital abnormality should be dismantled and no new ones established. Private prenatal testing should, of course, be allowed to continue.

4

Screening in the Independent Sector

IT is often argued that the private sector is poor at providing preventive medicine because much of it is a public good that everyone will benefit from if only one person will supply it. This may be true for clean air and water and mosquito control programmes, but most screening is a private good. People pay for it because it benefits either themselves or their family. So long as they can choose where they get it, providers have an incentive to offer it (Baker *et al* 1994, Showstack *et al* 1996). Laing's Review of Private Health Care 1995 (Laing and Buisson 1995) lists 177 private screening clinics in the UK, offering a wide range of services including most of the programmes described in chapter 3. These clinics have an estimated turnover on their screening activities of £31 million, which is modest compared with other areas of the independent medical sector, (curative medicine £1,700 million, long-term care £5,896 million, vision services £700 million, complementary medicine £500 million) but is rising. This relatively small amount of private activity suggests that unmet demand in the UK is largely for tests of disputed cost/benefit, or from people wanting extras, such as convenient clinic times, or access to a female doctor. Nevertheless, unless there is substantial over-provision in the NHS, private screening would probably rise dramatically if NHS screening were reduced.

In the United States, with a larger private health care sector and more private screening activity, doctors and patients tend to be particularly enthusiastic about screening. Doctors in 'fee-for-service' practice have more positive preventive beliefs, attitudes and practices, than those in health maintenance organisations (HMOs) (Scutchfield and de Moor 1989) and many American patients believe that almost all cancers can be screened for (Appenheimer 1987). Private patients were six times more likely to have had prostate-specific antigen screening than clinic patients (Perez and Tsou 1995) despite both clinics aiming to follow the same guidelines. The private patients were seven times more likely to have been screened in accordance with the guidelines. Private United States doctors almost invariably offer adult screening for hypertension, cholesterol and bowel cancer (Robbins *et al* 1993) often in health maintenance protocols (Hahn and Berger 1990), as well as offering women mammography, breast self-examination counselling, pelvic examination, and Pap smear (Clark *et al* 1995, Salive *et al* 1996). Besides immunisation, they often also offer children cholesterol screening (Bennet *et al* 1993). Enthusiasts offer ultrasound screening for ovarian cancer (Holbert 1994), cocaine screening in pregnancy (Burke and Roth 1993) and even screening for lead poisoning in children (Schenker *et al* 1994).

The difference between the United States and United Kingdom is not confined to programmes such as hypertension, cholesterol and cancer screening, where the low NHS rate is partly due to doubt about overall cost/benefit. The United States has consistently achieved higher child immunisation rates than the UK, mostly provided by private medicine (Yankauer 1983), supplemented by government programmes to ensure that the children of the poor are not neglected. It helps that children in America are not admitted to school without a certificate that they have been immunised. Managed care organisations in the United States are increasingly involved in population-based prevention activities. For example, the Group Health Association of America has published a list of best practices for preventive medicine and, with other managed care organisations, is committed to fully immunising at least 90 per cent of their enrolled children by two years of age (Gordon *et al* 1996). Other HMOs sponsor HIV prevention campaigns and youth violence prevention initiatives, sometimes targeted at the whole community, not just those enrolled in their plan (Gordon *et al* 1996). The Health Plan Employer Data and Information Set (HEDIS 2.0), developed with the independent National Committee on Quality Assurance, produces report cards for consumers indicating the extent to which HMOs such as the Henry Ford Health System, Harvard Pilgrim Health Care, Prudential,

United Health Care, and Kaiser Permante (Kaiser Permante 1995, Showstack *et al* 1996), have achieved selected public health targets including child immunisation rates.

Not surprisingly there is variation in screening provision by different health care plans and between different 'fee-for-service' doctors (Steiner *et al* 1997). If this occurred within the NHS, it would be a cause for concern. However, for an unproven technology where there are multiple private health care plans and 'fee-for-service' providers, it is a healthy sign of diversity which increases patient choice. In the long term such diversity helps everyone discover what is worthwhile (Herzlinger 1997).

Charity Screening

The voluntary sector is another source of independent screening (Harris 1996). Although most people agree that the poor should not have to depend on charity for curative care (Pinker 1996), the voluntary organisations are an adaptable, innovative and efficient way to supply screening of disputed cost/benefit. There are many examples in the US (Hart *et al* 1995, Reardon 1995). Nearly 8,000 optometrists are involved in the 'Vision USA' programme, which provides free eye examinations (Miller 1993) and other voluntary organisations are involved in mammography (Fink and Hutter (1987) and in cholesterol screening (Wynder *et al* 1986). Su Salud ('your health' in Spanish), a Californian charity which refuses to accept public funds, provides health screening, education and counselling, including blood pressure tests, immunisations, cholesterol screen, dental check-ups, glaucoma tests, PAP smears and pelvic and prostate examinations to uninsured Spanish speakers in an annual health fair. More than 3,000 volunteer health care workers are involved. In the UK there is less scope for charitable screening because of NHS provision, but the Marie Stopes clinics provide cervical screening free for those who cannot afford to pay.

US private health care programmes also offer low-cost or free screening for the poor (Sickles *et al* 1987, Bird 1987). For example, the Elderly Health Screening Service (EHSS) in Connecticut provides comprehensive annual health screening to people aged over 60 for a suggested donation of $20, or $25 with Pap testing. This includes blood cholesterol, urinalysis, electrocardiogram, blood pressure, faecal blood test, breast examination and instruction in self-examination, Pap test, digital prostate examination, vision, and hearing. Although such subsidised screening is presumably funded by loading the charges of other people who pay for private health care, this is not coercive in the way that state taxation is. If paying customers' fees are loaded too heavily, or loaded to fund programmes of which the customers disapprove, they are free to seek other insurance providers.

Two Futures

Here are my predictions of the future, with or without the state as the primary health-screening provider.

1. State Screening Continues

If the state goes on providing adult screening a steady expansion in provision will progressively erode individual liberty. Experts will choose how much to spend on screening and what programmes to choose. As they do so individuals will find it increasingly difficult to choose different programmes, or to save money on screening and spend it on curative care if they turn out to be unlucky. As the novelty wears off, screening will become a Cinderella service, with buildings falling into disrepair, the best staff leaving, and those that remain not bothering to explain what they are doing to patients. Clinic hours will become less convenient, and waiting times will increase, so that only the most motivated patients will turn up. Retraining and quality circles to remedy these problems will add layers of bureaucracy to already inefficient services. Patients will have no incentive to keep informed, since the decisions they could have made for themselves will have been removed. Planners will set up mobile and community clinics to encourage attendance. Before long someone will recommend financial incentives to encourage attendance by the recalcitrant poor (Dern *et al* 1994, Giuffrida and Torgerson 1997). Not only will people be forced to pay for poor quality screening, but they will also be forced to pay to persuade those who do not want it to turn up!

2. Screening Without the State

If the state withdrew from adult health screening, private clinics would continue to offer it. They would offer different tests, in different packages, at different costs. Some programmes would be cheap, because the providers skimped on the service aspect, offered cheaper tests, or limited the number of tests. The famous high street names, such as Virgin, Sainsbury and Marks and Spencer, would probably join in and advertise their services. Many tests would be offered for use by patients at home. Home pregnancy testing is already widespread and home HIV, faecal blood and drug monitoring tests are already available (Roberts 1996). When faced with all this choice, wise patients would seek advice from consumer organisations, screening brokers, or their general practitioner. Newspaper and magazine articles and the experience of friends and relatives would temper this advice. A more informed population would increasingly use information technology to participate in their own health care decision-making (Smith 1997, Jennings *et al* 1997). They would be educated not only in the technical aspects of the test, but in the principles of screening, interpretation of risk, and the effectiveness of interventions. Microsoft, consumer groups, chat groups and researchers, would probably provide information on the Internet. Ultimately the choices of educated patients in the screening market would select the worthwhile programmes that were commercially viable.

Like now, the poor would get less testing than the rich in such a world. However, in the long run they would probably get more and better testing than in the state-provided alternative. They would certainly get testing that followed their own priorities more closely. Providers would offer cheap introductory screening deals, both as a way of demonstrating their social conscience and as loss leaders to gain future customers, and charities would subsidise some tests, or offer them free. This would probably happen relatively soon with prenatal testing, because some people feel strongly about it.

5

What Should the NHS Do?

1. The NHS should not normally provide screening programmes for healthy adults. Private programmes would be both more efficient and more responsive to consumers, who are the only people able to judge whether the benefits outweigh the side-effects sufficiently to justify the cost. The three main adult NHS programmes, hypertension screening, mammography and cervical cytology, should be privatised, and those who wish to undergo such screening should pay for it.
2. The government should also make it clear that the NHS will not take on the provision of future similar screening programmes. There are many effective programmes which current public health orthodoxy judges not cost/beneficial but which some individuals nevertheless choose to undergo privately. Examples include cholesterol screening, prostate specific antigen, faecal occult blood, and ovarian cancer. These should remain the responsibility of the private health care sector.
3. The NHS should continue to provide screening of undisputed cost/benefit to adults who could not otherwise afford it, on the grounds that the state thereby alleviates poverty. No adult screening programmes for the general population presently fulfil this criteria, but some do when applied, either systematically or opportunistically, to high-risk groups. Examples include screening for tuberculosis among the homeless, for hyper-cholesterolaemia among relatives of people with early onset cardiovascular disease, and genetic screening for cancer susceptibility among relatives of sufferers.
4. The NHS should also continue to provide screening services where there are significant beneficial externalities that might otherwise cause the service to be priced too high privately. The main examples are screening for infectious disease, particularly TB and sexually transmitted disease.

5. The NHS should continue to provide effective screening services for children and the mentally impaired. Examples include new-born screening for phenyl-ketonuria and hypothyroidism. The justification is to protect them from avoidable harm by lazy or incompetent parents or carers.
6. For the same reasons the NHS should continue to provide prenatal screening where the aim is to improve the health of the baby. Examples include hypertension, rhesus, rubella and syphilis testing.
7. The NHS should stop supplying antenatal screening where the aim is to permit abortion of abnormal fetuses. This does not fulfil any of the criteria for state intervention in health care and has harmful externalities. Such screening should continue to be permitted privately.

How Can These Policies Be Implemented?

These policies are feasible because they do not involve depriving any sick individuals of a benefit that they believe to be rightfully theirs. NHS withdrawal from providing routine eye tests and dental care indicate that, when the 'rule of rescue' is not broken, it can be done. At the very least, health planners should not introduce new NHS programmes without evidence that the NHS will do better than the private sector. This means not only waiting for evidence of effectiveness, but also for private demand to demonstrate cost benefit, and for evidence that it provides a public good, improves externalities or helps children or the handicapped. Resisting calls for new government screening will be easier once the principle that adult screening is a private decision is established.

NHS withdrawal from prenatal screening for fetal abnormality will be more controversial, but is an even more important policy recommendation. Other NHS screening simply allocates resources badly, but NHS prenatal screening harms the living handicapped now, with the risk of worse to come in future, if politicians supporting eugenic policies ever came to power. Withdrawal would provide a line which politicians would find it difficult to cross, and be an important future safeguard. NHS screeners will argue that it will result in more handicapped children being born to poor families, but the force of their argument can always be blunted by reminding people that such collectivists would have preferred these children to have been killed instead. Liberal reformers will have two powerful allies, the 'pro-life' movement and those advocates of the disabled who recognise how current policies discriminate against them. Such an alliance should have the power to get the NHS out of this particular activity. Professional politicians will be wary of reopening the abortion issue as a party policy, and the initiative will probably come from a private members bill. The following might prove useful.

Some Sound Bites

- Whenever you hear the word 'free' substitute the word 'compulsory'. If something is provided 'free' to one person, someone else is 'forced' to pay for it.
- Screening tests are lottery tickets. Even the best cost everyone a bit of inconvenience and anxiety so that a few people can win big.
- Prenatal screening is a very risky lottery ticket. Although some people win the prize of preventing the birth of a handicapped child, others lose a healthy wanted pregnancy.
- We don't correct poverty by giving poor people lottery tickets that even the rich wouldn't buy.
- Why should people who think abortion is murder be forced to pay for programmes that encourage other people to kill their unborn babies?
- If someone offered you a tablet for £7,000, which would, on average, give you an extra year of life in full health, would you buy it? Cervical screening and mammography cost this much for each year of life gained, and are a lot less convenient than swallowing a tablet.
- Are older women deprived by not being invited for mammography? Those who want it can already get it free by just turning up. Only two per cent of older women bother.
- The NHS should still provide screening for fetuses, new-born babies, children and the handicapped. It should stop providing screening for healthy adults and screening which encourages abortion.

- Some government programmes are not just free. They pay poor people to encourage them to undergo screening.* Not only are taxpayers forced to pay for poor quality screening, but they are forced to pay to persuade those who do not want it to turn up!

---

* So far as I am aware this has not yet been tried in screening practice in the UK, but the idea is not too far fetched. The effect of such incentives is the subject of scientific study (Giufridda and Torgerson 1997). Taxi vouchers have been tried in the United States to encourage people to attend for prenatal screening (Melnokow *et al* 1997) and the French government persuades pregnant women to undergo toxoplasmosis testing by making it a requirement for maternity benefit.

Bibliography

Abelson, J. and Lomas J., 'Do health service organizations and community health centres have higher disease prevention and health promotion levels than fee-for-service practices?', *Canadian Medical Association Journal*, 142(6), 1990, pp. 575-81.

Adzick, N.S., Sutton, L.N., Cromblehome, T.M. and Flake, A.W., 'Successful fetal surgery for spina bifida', *Lancet*, 352, 1998, pp. 1675-76.

Anonymous, 'My mother's tormented death', *British Medical Journal*, 310, 1995, p. 67.

Anonymous, 'There's nothing I can do, I'm only a doctor', *British Medical Journal*, 314, 1997, pp. 759-60.

Appenheimer, A.T., 'Screening and diagnosis of cancer in office practice', *Primary Care: Clinics in Office Practice*, 14(2), 1987, pp. 255-69.

Arrow, K.J., 'Social choice and individual values', *Cowles Foundation Monograph*, 12, Yale University Press, 1963a.

Arrow, K.J., 'Uncertainty and the welfare economics of medical care', *American Economic Review*, 53, 1963b, pp. 941-73.

Audit Commission, *Fundholding: the Main Report*, London: Audit Commission, 1996.

Baker, E.L., Melton, R.J., Stange, P.V., Fields, M.L., Koplan, J.P., Guerra, F.A. and Satcher, D., 'Health reform and the health of the public. Forging community health partnerships', *Journal of the American Medical Association*, 272, 1994, pp. 1276-82.

Barron, C.M., 'There must be cost effective private health care', *British Medical Journal*, 313, 1996, pp. 1152-53.

Bekker, H., Modell, M., Dennis, G., Silver, A., Matthew, C., Bobrow, M. and Marteau, T., 'Uptake of cystic fibrosis testing in primary care: supply push or demand pull', *British Medical Journal*, 306, 1993, pp. 1584-86.

Bennett, M.J., Tershakovec, A.M., Cortner, J.A. and Shannon, B.M., 'A quality assurance program for the measurement of capillary blood cholesterol levels in private pediatric practices. The Children's Health Project', *American Journal of Diseases of Children*, 147, 1993, pp. 340-45.

Bentley, J.M., Green, P. and Ship, I.I., 'Achieving health outcomes through professional dental care: comparing the costs of dental treatment for children in three practice modes', *Health Services Research*, 19, 1984, pp. 181-96.

Bernstein, A.B., Thompson, G.B. and Harlan, L.C., 'Differences in rates of cancer screening by usual source of medical care. Data from the 1987 National Health Interview Survey', *Medical Care*, 29(3), 1991, pp. 196-209.

Berwick, D.M. and Weinstein, M.C., 'What do patients value? Willingness to pay for ultrasound in normal pregnancy', *Medical Care*, 23, 1985, pp. 881-93.

Bird, R.E., 'A successful effort to lower costs in screening mammography', *Cancer*, 60, 1987, pp. 1684-87.

Bordley, W.C., Margolis, P.A. and Lannon, C.M., 'The delivery of immunizations and other preventive services in private practices', *Pediatrics*, 97, 1996, pp. 467-73.

Brambati, B., Cislaghi, C., Tului, L., Alberti, E., Amidani, M., Colombo, U. and Zuliani, G., 'First-trimester Down's syndrome screening using nuchal translucency: a prospective study in patients undergoing chorionic villus sampling', *Ultrasound in Obstetrics & Gynecology*, 5, 1995, pp. 9-14.

Britchford, B., 'Grime and punishment', *British Medical Journal*, 311, 1996, p. 1098.

Brown, J., Melincovitch, P., Gitteman, B., Ricketts, S., 'Missed opportunities in preventive pediatric health care. Immunizations or well child care visits', *American Journal of Diseases of Children*, 147, 1993, pp.1081-84.

Burke, M.S. and Roth, D., 'Anonymous cocaine screening in a private obstetric population', *Obstetrics & Gynecology*, 81, 1993, pp. 354-56.

Clarke, A., 'Is non directive genetic counselling possible?', *Lancet*, 338, 1991, pp. 998-1001.

Clark, R., Geller, B., Peluso, N., McVety, D. and Worden, J.K., 'Development of a community mammography registry: experience in the breast screening program project', *Radiology*, 196, 1995, pp. 811-15.

Cohen, M.M., Roos, N.P., MacWilliam, L. and Wajda, A., 'Assessing physicians' compliance with guidelines for Papanicolaou testing', *Medical Care*, 30(6), June 1992, pp. 514-28.

Crick, R.P. and Tuck, M.W., 'How can we improve the detection of glaucoma?', *British Medical Journal*, 310, 1995, pp.546-47.

Cuckburn, J., Staples, M., Hurley, S. and de Juise, T., 'Psychological costs of screening mammography', *Journal of Medical Screening,* 1, 1994, pp. 7-12.

Cuckle, H.S., Wald, N.J., in Wald. N.J. (ed.), *Antenatal and Neonatal Screening*, Oxford: Oxford University Press, 1984.

Cuckle, H.S., 'Breast cancer screening by mammography: an overview', *Clinical Radiology*, 43, 1991, pp. 77-80.

Cuckle, H.S. *et al,* 'Fragile X', *Journal of Medical Screening*, 4, 1997, pp. 60-94.

Culyer, A., 'Needs – is a consensus possible?' *Journal of Medical Ethics,* 24, 1998, pp.77-80.

Davies, T., 'The view from the queue', *British Medical Journal*, 312, 1996, p. 1548.

Dern, S., Stephens, R., Davis, W.R., Feucht, T.E. and Tortu, S., 'The impact of providing incentives for attendance at AIDS prevention sessions', *Public Health Reports*, 109, 1994, pp. 548-54.

Devlin, B., Hanham, I., Le Fanu, J., Lefever, R., Mantell, B. and Freeman, M., *Medical Care: Is It a Consumer Good?*, Health Unit paper no. 8, London: IEA, 1990.

Diamond, P., 'Organising the health insurance market', *Econometrica*, 60, 1992, pp. 1233-54.

Doherty, N., Horowitz, D.A. and Crakes, G., 'Real costs of dental care in private and public practices', *Medical Care,* 18, 1980, pp. 96-109.

Donaldson, C., 'Willingness to pay for publicly-provided goods: a possible measure of benefit?', *Journal of Health Economics*, 9, 1990, pp. 103-18.

Donelan, K. *et al*, 'All payer, single payer, managed care, no payer: patients' perspectives in three nations', *Health Affairs*, 15, 1996, pp. 254-65.

Drummond, M.F., Stoddart, G.L. and Torrance, G.W., *Methods of Economic Evaluation in Health Care Programmes*, Oxford: Oxford University Press, 1987.

Dunlop, M. and Campbell, H., 'Screening for people with a family history of colorectal cancer', *British Medical Journal*, 314, 1997, pp. 1779-80.

Dworkin, R.M., *Life's Dominion: An Argument About Abortion and Euthanasia*, London: Harper Collins, 1995.

Epstein, K.A., Schneiderman, L.J., Bush, J.W. *et al*, 'The abnormal screening of serum thyroxine (T4): analysis of physician response, outcome, cost and health effectiveness', *Journal of Chronic Diseases*, 34, 1981, pp. 175-90.

Family Heart Study Group, 'Randomised controlled trial evaluating cardiovascular risk screening and intervention in general practice: principal results of British family heart study', *British Medical Journal*, 308, 1994, pp. 313-20.

Farizo, K.M., Stehr-Green, P.A., Markovitz, L.E., Patriarca, P.A. *et al*, 'Vaccination levels and missed opportunities for measles vaccination: a record audit in a public paediatric clinic', *Pediatrics*, 89, 1992, pp. 598-92.

Fink, D. and Hutter, R., 'Voluntary organisations in screening mammography', *Cancer*, 60, 1987, p. 1697.

Forss, H. and Widstrom, E., 'Factors influencing the selection of restorative materials in dental care in Finland', *Journal of Dentistry*, 24, 1996, pp. 257-62.

Frame, P.S., Kowulich, B.A. and Llewellyn, A.M., 'Improving physician compliance with a health maintenance protocol', *Journal of Family Practice*, 19(3), 1984, pp. 341-44.

Freemantle, N., Barbour, R., Johnson, R., Marchment, M. and Kennedy, A., 'The use of statins: a case of misleading priorities?', *British Medical Journal*, 315, 1997, pp. 826-28.

Giuffrida, A. and Torgerson, D., 'Should we pay the patient? Review of financial incentives to enhance patient compliance', *British Medical Journal*, 315, 1997, pp. 703-06.

Gordon, R., Baker, E., Roper, W. and Omenn, G., 'Prevention and the reforming US health care system: changing roles and responsibilities', *Annual Review of Public Health*, 17, 1996, pp. 489-509.

Gould, S.G., *The Mismeasure of Man*, London: Penguin, 1983.

Gredler, B. and Gerstner, G.J., 'Value of breast palpation in gynecologic practice', original title, 'Stellenwert der brustpalpation in der gynakologischen praxis', *Wiener Medizinische Wochenschrift*, 137(16), 1987, pp. 388-90.

Green, D.G. (ed.), Brown P., Burstall, M.L., Mossialos, E., Redwood, H. and Reekie, W.D., *Should Pharmaceutical Prices be Regulated?*, London: IEA Health and Welfare Unit, 1997.

Griffiths, P.G., 'A surfeit of screening?', British Medical Journal, 315, 1997, p. 318.

Hadorn, D.C., 'Setting health care priorities in Oregon. Cost effectiveness meets the rule of rescue', *Journal of the American Medical Association*, 265, 1991, pp. 2218-25.

Hahn, D.L. and Berger, M.G., 'Implementation of a systematic health maintenance protocol in a private practice', *Journal of Family Practice*, 31(5), 1990, pp. 492-502.

Hansagi, H., Calltorp, J. and Andreasson, S., 'Quality comparisons between privately and publicly managed health care centres in a suburban area of Stockholm, Sweden', *Quality Assurance in Health Care*, 5, 1993, pp. 33-40.

Hakama, M., Chamberlain, J., Day, N.E., Miller, A.B. and Prorok, P.C., 'Evaluation of screening programmes for gynaecological cancer', *British Journal of Cancer*, 52, 1985, pp. 669-73.

Harris, J.R., Gordon, R.L., White, K.E., Stange, P.V. and Harper, S.M., 'Prevention and managed care; opportunities for managed care organisations, purchasers of health care and public health agencies', *Journal of the American Medical Association*, 275, 1996, pp. 26-29.

Hart, J.T., 'The inverse care law', *Lancet*, i, 1971, pp. 495-503.

Hart, P.L., Wood, C.B. and Pupecki, M.A., 'Private sector volunteerism as a solution to caring for the uninsured', *Journal of the American Medical Association*, 273, 1995, p. 1487.

Haynes, R.B., Sackett, D.L., Taylor, D.W., Gibson, E.S. and Johnson, A.L., 'Increased absenteeism from work after detection and labelling of hypertensive patients', *New England Journal of Medicine,* 299, 1978, pp.741-44.

Health Departments of Great Britain, 'General Practice in the National Health Service: the 1990 contract', 1989.

HEDIS 2.0 (Health plan Employer Data and Information Set): Executive Summary, Washington DC: National Committee for Quality Assurance, 1993.

Herzlinger, R.E., *Market-driven Healthcare*, Reading, Massachusetts: Addison-Wesley Publishing Co., 1997.

Holbert, T.R., 'Screening transvaginal ultrasonography of postmenopausal women in a private office setting', *American Journal of Obstetrics & Gynecology*, 170, 1994, pp.1699-703; discussion pp.1703-04.

Holland, W.W., Stewart, S., *Screening in Health Care: Benefit or Bane*, London: Nuffield Provincial Hospitals Trust, 1990.

Imperial Cancer Research Fund OXCHECK Study Group, 'Effectiveness of health checks conducted by nurses in primary care: final results of the Oxcheck study', *British Medical Journal*, 310, 1995, pp. 1099-104.

Jacoby, A., McCann, K., 'Gaps exist between policy and reality', *British Medical Journal*, 310, 1995, p. 1204.

Jennings, K., Miller, K. and Materna, S., *Changing Health Care*, Santa Monica: Knowledge Exchange, 1997.

Johnstone, M.F., Gibson, S., Wayne, T.C., Haynes, R.B., Taylor, D.W., Gafni, A. and Sincurella, J., 'Effects of labelling on income work and social function among hypertensive employees', *Journal of Chronic Diseases*, 37, 1984, pp. 417-23.

Joint National Committee on Detection, 'Evaluation and treatment of high blood pressure', fifth report of the JNCDETHBP (JNC V), *Archives of Internal Medicine*, 153, 1993, pp. 154-83.

Judge, K., 'Value for money in the British residential care industry', in Culyer, A.J. and Jonsson, B. (eds.), *Public and Private Health Services: Complementarities and Conflicts*, Oxford: Blackwell, 1986.

Juniper, M., 'The tale of two wards', *British Medical Journal*, 313, 1996, p. 1152.

Kaiser Permante 1993 Quality Report Card, Oakland California: Kaiser Permante 1993.

Kelsell, D.P., Dunlop, J., Stevens, H.P. *et al*, 'Connexin 26 mutations in heriditary non-syndromic sensorineural deafness', *Nature*, 16, 1997, pp. 188-90.

Knapp, M. 'The relative cost-effectiveness of public, voluntary and private providers of residential child care', in Culyer, A.J., Jonsson, B. (eds.), *Public and Private Health Services: Complementarities and Conflicts*, Oxford: Blackwell, 1986.

Krahn, M.D., Mahoney, J.E., Eckman, M.H., Trachtenberg, J., Pauker, S.G., Detsky, A.S., 'Screening for prostate cancer: a decision analytic view', *Journal of the American Medical Association*, 272, 1994, pp. 773-80.

Laidlaw, D.A.H., Bloom, P.A., Hughes, A.O., Sparrow, J.M. and Marmion, V.J., 'The sight test fee: effect on ophthalmology referrals and rate of glaucoma detection', *British Medical Journal*, 309, 1994,pp. 634-36.

Laing and Buisson, *Laing's Review of Private Healthcare 1995*, London: Laing and Buisson, 1995.

Lantz, P.M., Weigers, M.E., House, J.S., 'Education and income differentials in breast and cervical cancer screening. Policy implications for rural women', *Medical Care*, 35, 1997, pp. 219-36.

Leff, A.M., Berger, R., Lotspeich, E. and Dillard, C.O., (1977) 'Private practice in the public sector: a unique relationship among local government, physicians, and health care consumers in Cincinnati', *Medical Care*, 15(10), 1977, pp. 838-48.

Letters, 'Use of statins', *British Medical Journal*, 315, 1997, pp. 1615-20.

Lilford, R.J. and Thornton, J.G., 'Prenatal screening vouchers', *Journal of the Royal Society of Medicine*, 89, 1995, pp. 130-31.

Mansley, C. 'My 27-year wait for an NHS diagnosis', *British Medical Journal*, 313, 1996, p. 1014.

Mason, J., Drummond, M. and Torrance, G., 'Some guidelines on the use of cost-effectiveness league tables', British Medical Journal, 306, 1993, pp. 570-72.

Maynard, A., 'Developing the health care market', *The Economic Journal*, 101, 1991, pp. 1277-86.

McConnachie, K.M. and Roghmann, K.J., 'Immunisation opportunities missed among urban poor children', *Pediatrics*, 89, 1992, pp. 1019-26.

Melnokow, J., Paliescheskey, M. and Stewart, G.K., 'Effect of a transportation incentive on compliance with the first prenatal appointment: a randomised trial', *Obstetrics and Gynecology*, 89, 1997, pp. 1023-27.

Middleton, A., Hewison, J. and Mueller, R.F., 'Attitudes of deaf adults toward genetic testing for hereditary deafness', *American Journal of Human Genetics*, 63, 1998, p. 1175-80.

Miller, S.C., 'VISION USA: optometry's national charity program', *Journal of the American Optometric Association*, 64, 1993, pp. 613-16.

Muldoon, M.F. and Criqui, M.H., 'The emerging role of statins in the prevention of coronary heart disease', *British Medical Journal*, 315, 1997, pp. 1554-55.

NHS Centre for Reviews and Dissemination, 'Screening for prostate cancer', *Effectiveness Matters*, 2, 1997.

Nutting, P.A., Burkhalter, B.R., Dietrick, D.L. and Helmick, E.F., 'Relationship of size and payment mechanism to system performance', *Medical Care*, 20, 1982, pp. 676-90.

Office of National Statistics, 'Abortion statistics, AB No. 23', London: The Government Statistical Service, 1996.

Office of National Statistics, 'Mortality statistics, DH2 No. 22', London: The Government Statistical Service, 1996.

Orme, R., 'Pitching it low', *British Medical Journal*, 312, 1996, p. 1486.

Perez, N., Tsou, H.H., 'Prostate cancer screening practices: differences between clinic and private patients', *Mount Sinai Journal of Medicine*, 62, 1995, pp. 316-21.

Pinker, R., 'Falling back on charity', *British Medical Journal*, 313, 1996, p. 1566.

Pollitt, R., 'Tandem mass spectrometry screening in the new-born', *Health Technology Assessment*, 1(7), 1997.

Reardon, R.M., 'Private sector volunteerism as a solution to caring for the uninsured', *Journal of the American Medical Association*, 273, 1995, p. 1487.

Reardon, W., 'Connexin 26 gene mutation and autosomal recessive deafness', *Lancet*, 351, 1998, pp.383-84.

Reynolds, F., 'Are hospital patients fellow human beings?', *British Medical Journal,* 312, 1996, pp. 982-83.

Robbins, J.A., Dickinson, W.A., Bartel, A.G. and Hartman, C.W., 'Lipid management program: results of applying national guidelines in a private practice', *Southern Medical Journal*, 86, 1993, pp. 289-92.

Roberts, J., 'Controversy surrounds home monitoring and diagnosis', *British Medical Journal,* 313, 1996, p. 1354.

Rosser, R., Kind, P. and Williams, A., 'Valuation of quality of life: some psychometric evidence', in Jones-Lee, M. (ed.), *The Value of Life and Society*, Amsterdam: Elsevier, 1982.

Sackett, D.L. and Torrance, G.W., 'The utility of different health states as perceived by the public', *Journal of Chronic Diseases*, 31, 1978, pp. 697-704.

Salive, M.E., Guralnik, J.M. and Brock, D., 'Preventive services for breast and cervical cancer in US office-based practices', *Preventive Medicine*, 25, 1996, pp. 561-68.

Schenker, T.L., Fritz, C.J., Murphy, A. and Shepeard, S., 'Feasibility and effectiveness of screening for childhood lead poisoning in private medical practice', *Archives of Pediatrics & Adolescent Medicine*, 148, 1994, pp. 761-64.

Scutchfield, F.D. and de Moor, C., 'Preventive attitudes, beliefs, and practices of physicians in fee-for-service and health maintenance organization settings', *Western Journal of Medicine*, 150(2), 1989, pp. 221-25.

Seeman, M. and Seeman, T., 'Health behaviour and personal autonomy: a longitudinal study of the sense of control in illness', *Journal of Health and Social Behaviour*, 24, 1983, pp.144-60.

Showstack, J., Luie, N., Leatherman, S., Fisher, E. and Inui, T., 'Health of the public. The private sector challenge', *Journal of the American Medical Association*, 276, 1996, pp. 1071-74.

Sickles, E.A., Weber, W.N., Galvin, H.B., Ominsky, S.H. and Sollitto, R.A., 'Low-cost mammography screening', *Cancer*, 60, 1987, pp. 1688-91.

Simpson, D.M., Suarez, L. and Smith, D.R., 'Immunization rates among young children in the public and private health care sectors', *American Journal of Preventive Medicine*, 13, 1997, pp. 84-88.

Sintonen, H., 'Comparing the productivity of public and private dentistry', in Culyer, A.J. and Jonsson, B. (eds.), *Public and Private Health Services: Complementarities and Conflicts*, Oxford: Blackwell 1986.

Smith, R., 'The future of healthcare systems. Information technology and consumerism will transform healthcare worldwide', *British Medical Journal*, 314, 1997, pp. 1495-96.

Smith, W.C.S., Lee, A.J., Crombie, I.K. and Tunstall-Pedoe, H., 'Control of blood pressure in Scotland: the rule of halves', British Medical Journal, 300, 1990, pp. 918-23.

Snowdon, S.K. and Stewart-Brown, S.L., *Pre-school Vision Screening: Results of a Systematic Review*, York: NHS Centre for Reviews and Dissemination, 1997.

Stenson, W.B. and Weinstein, M.C., 'Allocation of resources to manage hypertension', *New England Journal of Medicine,* 296, 1977, pp. 732-39.

Steiner, C.A., Powe, N.R., Anderson, G.F. and Das, A., 'Technology coverage decisions by health care plans and considerations by medical directors', *Medical Care*, 35, 1997, pp. 472-89.

Stewart-Brown, S. and Farmer, A., 'Screening could seriously damage your health', *British Medical Journal*, 314, 1997, pp. 533-34.

Stewart-Brown. S., Gillam, S. and Jewell, T., 'The problems of fundholding. Some benefits to patients but no effect on how doctors practise', *British Medical Journal*, 312, 1996, pp. 1311-12.

Sutton, G.C., 'Will you still need me, will you still screen me, when I'm past 64? Breast screening policy is based on ageism', *British Medical Journal*, 315, 1997, pp. 1032-33.

Szilagyi, P.G., Rodewall, L.E., Humiston, S.G. *et al,* (1993) 'Missed opportunities for childhood vaccinations in office practices and the effect on vaccination status', *Pediatrics*, 91, 1993, pp. 1-7.

Szilagyi, P.G., Roghmann, K.J., Campbell, J.R., Humiston, S.G., Winter, N.L., Raubertas, R.F. and Rodewald, L.E., 'Immunization practices of primary care practitioners and their relation to immunization levels', *Archives of Pediatrics and Adolescent Medicine*, 148,1994, pp. 158-66.

Thornton, J.G., 'Prenatal screening programmes', *Lancet*, ii, 1994, pp. 1090-91.

Thornton, J.G. and Lilford, R.J., 'Decision analysis for medical managers', *British Medical Journal*, 310, 1995, pp. 791-94.

Thornton, J.G., Hewison, J., Lilford, R.J. and Vail, A. 'A randomised trial of three methods of giving information about prenatal testing', *British Medical Journal*, 311, 1995, pp. 1127-30.

Torrance, G.W. and Zipursky, A. (1984) 'Cost-effectiveness of antepartum prevention of Rh immunization', *Clinics in Perinatology,*11, 1984, pp. 267-81.

Tymstra, T., 'False positive results on screening tests: experiences of parents of children screened for congenital hypothyroidism', *Family Practitioner,* 3, 1986, pp. 92-96.

Tymstra, T. and Bielman, B., (1987) 'The psychosocial impact of mass screening for disease', *Family Practitioner,* 4, 1987, pp. 287-90.

USPTF, United States Preventive Services Task Force, *Guide to Clinical Preventive Services*, Second edition, Baltimore: Williams and Wilkins, 1996.

Wakeham, A.P. and Leach, R.H., 'Health authorities must work with clinicians to target statins', *British Medical Journal*, 315, 1997, p. 1618.

Wald, N.J., 'Screening brief: breast cancer', *Journal of Medical Screening*, i, 1994, p. 73.

Wenham, P., 'Bureaucracy gone mad', *British Medical Journal*, 313, 1996, p. 949.

Wisconsin Cystic Fibrosis Neonatal Screening Group, 'Nutritional benefits of neonatal screening for cystic fibrosis', *New England Journal of Medicine,* 337, 1997, pp. 963-69.

Williams, G.A., Abbott, R.R. and Taylor, D.K., 'Using focus group methodology to develop breast cancer screening programs that recruit African American women', *Journal of Community Health*, 22, 1997, pp. 45-56.

Wilson, J.M.G. and Jungner, G., *Principles and Practice of Screening for Disease*, Geneva: World Health Organisation, 1968.

Wise, J., 'British public supports legal abortion for all', *British Medical Journal*, 314, 1997, p. 627.

Wonderling, D., Langham, S., Buxton, M., Normand, C. and McDermott, C., 'What can be concluded from the OXCHECK and British family heart studies: commentary on cost effectiveness analyses', *British Medical Journal*, 312, 1996, pp. 1274-78.

Working Group on Acute Purchasing, *Statin therapy / HNG CoA Reductase Inhibitor Treatment in the Prevention of Coronary Heart Disease*, Sheffield: Trent Institute for Health Services Research, University of Sheffield, 1996.

Wormald, R., Fraser, S. and Bunce, C., 'Time to look again at sight tests', *British Medical Journal*, 314, 1997, p. 245.

Wynder, E.L., Field, F. and Haley, N.J., 'Population screening for cholesterol determination. A pilot study', *Journal of the American Medical Association*, 256, 1986, pp. 2839-42.

Yankauer, A., 'Public and private prevention', *American Journal of Public Health*, 73, 1983, pp. 1032-34.

Yates, J., *Private Eye, Heart and Hip*, Edinburgh: Churchill Livingstone, 1995.

IEA Health and Welfare Unit

Independence

The Health and Welfare Unit is part of the Institute of Economic Affairs, a registered educational charity (No. 235351) founded in 1955. Like the IEA, the Health and Welfare Unit is financed from a variety of private sources to avoid over-reliance on any single or small group of donors.

All IEA publications are independently refereed and referees' comments are passed on anonymously to authors. The IEA gratefully acknowledges the contributions made to its educational work by the eminent scholars who act as referees.

All the Institute's publications seek to further its objective of promoting the advancement of learning, by research into economic and political science, by education of the public therein, and by the dissemination of ideas, research and the results of research in these subjects. The views expressed are those of the authors, not of the IEA, which has no corporate view.